STRICTLY ANONYMOUS

Confessions

SECRET SEX LIVES
OF TOTAL STRANGERS

STRICTLY ANONYMOUS *Confessions*

SECRET SEX LIVES OF TOTAL STRANGERS

BY
KATHY KAY

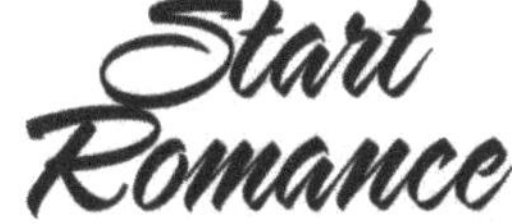

Published in the United States by Start Romance, an imprint of
Start Publishing, LLC, 221 River Street, Ninth Floor,
Hoboken, New Jersey 07030.

Printed in the United States
Cover design: Paula Guran
Cover image: Shutterstock/SALMAN HOSSAIN SOHEL & Rick Mullenix,
Mullenix Design, LLC
Text design: Westchester Publishing Services

First Edition.
10 9 8 7 6 5 4 3 2 1

Trade paper ISBN: 978-1-62778-339-2
E-book ISBN: 978-1-62778-498-6

CONTENTS

FOREWORD

What is *my* secret life? What do *I* do behind closed doors? I've been anonymously hosting a successful podcast called *Strictly Anonymous Confessions* for over a decade. No one, except for a few close family members and friends, knows this.

I launched my show in 2013, when very few people were podcasting. I worked in entertainment at the time and one of my close comedian friends, who was also a podcaster, knew I liked to talk and suggested I start my own show. Since I had always secretly wanted to be a therapist, I decided to try out a call-in advice show—kind of like a modern-day *Dear Abby.*

The truth is I *do* talk a lot, but at least it's not about myself. What I really enjoy most is talking to other people. I love hearing their life stories, analyzing their problems, and offering my insight and opinions in return. But not everyone wants to talk about their personal issues, nor do they want help with them. Most of my friends were annoyed by my prying and they didn't want my input. I needed to find people who not only wanted to tell me their stories, but those who were open to hearing my advice.

And how exactly did I find those people? It was 2013—Facebook was one of the few social media platforms available and I didn't want to post there. My profile, much like everyone else's, was full of friends, family members, and coworkers—people who I didn't want knowing about the show. The truth is, I was 100 percent convinced that my show was going to tank, and I didn't want to suck in front of anyone I knew.

So, I decided to place an ad on Craigslist, in the only free section, which happened to be the personals. I posted the ad in every single subcategory including "casual encounters." It read:

> *Do you have a problem and need advice? Or do you live a secret life that you can't talk to anyone about and you want to come clean? If so,* The Strictly Anonymous *podcast would love to have you on the next show.*
>
> *We're looking for real people, with real problems who need advice or need to get something off their chest. Nothing is off limits, you remain completely anonymous and anything goes.*

Within hours of posting it, I received emails from five different guys with some of the craziest stories I had ever heard. One guy was screwing his best friend's brother-in-law, who happened to be the town's sheriff; another guy who could only get off when going down on women; and another who enjoyed watching his wife hook up with other men.

I booked them all right away. Since most of the men were going to be talking about what they were doing on the down-low, I decided it would be best to keep them anonymous. They all used fake names and altered voices to render them unrecognizable. I also made up a phony name for myself.

I taped those five guys all in the same day, and their stories became my first five episodes. It was also on that day that I came up with the name of my podcast—the rest is history. Craigslist really was the gift that kept on giving and thankfully, by the time

Craigslist personals went bust, the podcast was up and running and people kept emailing me to be on the show. Twelve years later, the podcast consists of more than one thousand episodes.

After talking to so many people, what I've come to realize, and what I want people to know, is that no matter how bizarre they sound, these are real stories about real people. Regular people who lead regular lives. This is just what they're doing behind closed doors. There is no "pervert island" where these "types of people" that do these "types of things," live. They don't look any different than anyone else because they're not different from anyone else. These people are your neighbors, your coworkers, your boss, your relatives, your best friend, or maybe even *you*?!

I've talked to people with all kinds of fetishes—women who love gang bangs, couples in open marriages, cucks and the hot wives they're married to, the bulls who fuck them as well as straight guys who sometimes like to suck a dick. You name it, I've talked about it on my show.

I believe that speaking openly about these types of things helps to "normalize" them, and I get daily emails from listeners thanking me for it. Though some people tune in for entertainment and some for education, a lot listen because knowing that there are other people out there who have the same kinks, fetishes, and interests as they do, makes them feel more "normal."

And what is *normal*? Normal is whatever people are really doing.

What are people *really* doing?? Well probably a lot more than they're actually telling you. But they do tell me, and that's what my show and this book are all about.

You're going to hear stories you've probably never heard before, but they're all true and I hope you enjoy them. I handpicked each one because it stood out to me in one way or another. These are some of the best, but there are over a thousand more on my podcast, *Strictly Anonymous Confessions.*

**Each story is based on an episode that has previously aired on my podcast. If you want to hear these stories told by the person themselves, you can! At the end of each story, I've listed the episode number, title, and link for you to check out.*

SEXXXY TERMS YOU NEED TO KNOW

Provided by SDC.com, the world's largest international, open-minded dating site for couples and singles.

Adult Arcade A store that has private booths where one can pay to view live or filmed adult content.

Adult Only Content reserved for adults who are twenty-one plus. The term usually describes parties, travel events, cruises, and resorts.

Adult Theaters Theaters that screen porn to viewers who are twenty-one plus. Audience members are allowed to masturbate, or hook up with other theater patrons.

Airtight When a woman (with consent) is simultaneously penetrated in her pussy, ass, and mouth.

Bathhouses A public bathhouse or sauna where people (usually gay men) can meet and have casual sexual encounters on-site.

BBC Big Black Cock (refers to genitals and a genre of porn).

BDSM Bondage, Discipline, Sadism, and Masochism.

Bi-Curious A heterosexual person who is curious about exploring things sexually with someone of the same gender.

Bisexual / Bi A person who is physically and/or emotionally attracted to their own gender as well as others.

Bull A man who (with consent) takes sexual ownership of another man's female partner (known as a hotwife or vixen).

Butt Plug a.k.a. Anal Plug, is a type of sex toy that is inserted into a person's ass.

CFNM Clothed Female Naked (or Nude) Male, which is a sexual fetish in which the female is clothed but the male is not.

Cisgender A person who identifies with the same gender they were assigned at birth.

Cock Cage A chastity device that prevents a man's cock from being stimulated/getting a full erection.

Compersion A person's emotional satisfaction of knowing and/or seeing the pleasure that their partner experiences with other people sexually and/or emotionally.

Consensual Nonconsent A BDSM scene involving role-playing as a person who is consensually forced into sex by an aggressor or a group of aggressors.

Cougar An older woman who enjoys prowling for younger play partners (of legal age and consenting).

Creampie A sex act that involves a man ejaculating into a pussy or ass (anal creampie) and then watching it leak.

Cross-Dresser / Cross-Dressing When a man gets a thrill out of dressing up in "feminine" clothing, like a dress, pantyhose, high heels, makeup, etc. (can sometimes be considered a kink or fetish).

Cross Swords When two men's cocks touch in threesomes or group sex scenarios.

Cruising When men drive or walk around at a location looking for other men to have sex with (often anonymous and a one-time encounter).

Cub A younger man, typically under thirty years old, who is romantically or sexually involved with an older woman.

Cuck / Cuckold / Cuckolding A man who wants to watch his female partner have sex with another man (or several men) without his direct involvement.

Cuckquean The female version of a cuckold. A woman who enjoys watching her man have sex with other women.

Doggy-Style A sex position where someone is fucked from behind while on all fours.

Dominant / Domming / Dom / Domme Dominance can be physical and/or psychological. This is performed by the Dominant (a.k.a., Dom/Domme or Master/Mistress or Top) on the submissive (a.k.a., sub or slave or bottom).

DP (Double Penetration) When a woman's pussy and ass are penetrated at the same time during sex.

Dungeon A room or area where people go to engage in BDSM (not always located underground).

DVP (Double Vaginal Penetration) When a woman is simultaneously penetrated with two phalluses (toy and/or cock).

Exhibitionism / Exhibitionist A person who gets aroused by being watched while nude and/or during sex.

Feminization a.k.a. sissification. A sexual fetish where a man reverses traditional gender roles while cross-dressing, sometimes during BDSM scenarios when he is submissive to a Domme/Dom/Dominant.

Fetish In kink terms, fetishes exist when a person is sexually aroused by a nonsexual object, piece of clothing, actions, and/or nongenital anatomy.

Fisting When a person inserts their entire hand, ideally in the form of a fist, into a pussy or an ass.

Flogging A harsh beating with a leather strap, whip, or rope, etc. Typically used in BDSM.

FMF (female-male-female) A threesome involving one male and two females in which the two females don't usually hook up.

Gag A device/sex toy that is inserted in a person's mouth to prevent them from talking during sex.

Gang bang When several people take turns fucking the same person.

GILF A "grandma I'd like to fuck."

Glory Holes A hole in a wall through which blow jobs, sex, or masturbation can be performed anonymously.

Hard Swap a.k.a. Full Swap. When two couples swap partners and fuck.

Hog-tie / Hog-tying Tying up someone's wrists and ankles with ropes or cuffs behind their back.

Hotel Takeover When a hotel venue is booked for a swingers-only party. It can include erotic events and designated rooms for play areas.

Hotwife / Hotwifing When a woman/female-identified person (the hotwife) has sex with other men with the full permission and encouragement from her partner.

Humiliation A consensual act wherein the feeling of embarrassment can evoke erotic excitement and/or sexual arousal.

Impact Play When a Dominant uses whips, crops, paddles, floggers, and/or other implements on a submissive's body in order to discipline, stimulate, and/or subdue them.

Kink Sexual practices that fall outside of cultural "norms." A kink is distinct from a fetish in that a kink is a *want*, and a fetish is a *need*.

Lesbian A female who is physically and emotionally attracted to other females.

Lifestyle Frequently called "The Lifestyle." Usually refers to the open, swinging, or kink communities and lifestyles.

Masochist A person who gets sexually aroused when receiving consensual physical or psychological pain that is inflicted by another person (usually the Dominant).

MFF (male-female-female) A threesome involving one male and two females. The two females hook up with each other, as well as hook up with the guy.

MFM (male-female-male) A threesome with two males and one female, in which the two males don't hook up.

MILF A "mom I'd like to fuck."

Mistress See Dominant.

Newbie Couples and singles who are new to the lifestyle.

NSA (No Strings Attached) Usually used to describe casual sexual interactions or hookups.

Orgasm Control a.k.a. Orgasm Denial. A sexual activity wherein someone's orgasm is denied or delayed for the purposes of enhancing sexual arousal.

Orgy When multiple people in the same room have sex with each other simultaneously.

Paddling When a Dominant uses a paddle tool on their submissive to provoke pleasurably painful sensations.

Peg / Pegged / Pegging A sexual practice where a woman anally penetrates a man with a strap-on dildo.

Play Partner A person with whom one has a casual sexual relationship.

Poly / Polyamory / Polyamorous Polyamory is a type of open relationship style and/or orientation in which a person is emotionally involved with more than one partner at the same time.

Reclaiming Sex Sex between a couple after one or both partners have consensually fucked someone else.

Rope Bondage Using rope to tie a person up. Frequently used during BDSM play.

Shibari A Japanese form of rope bondage. Very intricate and stylized.

Spit Roasting When a woman has a cock in her pussy and mouth at the same time.

Squirting Female ejaculation during sex.

Stag A man who encourages his female partner, known as a vixen, to have sex with other men. The stag, unlike the cuck, is *always* present when his hotwife has sex with another guy.

Submissive / Sub An individual who consensually gives another person the power to dominate them sexually and/or psychologically.

Swapping When couples trade partners for sexual play.

Swinger A person involved in the swinging lifestyle; see "Swinging."

Swinger Club A club/establishment specifically intended for couples and singles to meet and engage in on-premise sex.

Swinger House Parties Swinger events that are hosted at a private house or rented space.

Swinging The nonmonogamous pursuit of sexual partnerships with other individuals and couples.

Taint A slang term that refers to the perineum, an erogenous zone located between the asshole and the balls or pussy.

Threesome When three people engage in sexual activity with each other.

Throuple Three people who are in a sexual and romantic relationship with each other.

Train To "run a train" on someone is a term used during gang-bangs or group sex where one person receives penetration one or more at a time from multiple other people while others wait their turn in line.

Transgender A person who does not feel that their emotions, body, psychological comforts, and/or preferences are aligned with the gender they were assigned at birth.

Unicorn A single female who is open to playing with couples for threesomes.

Vanilla Someone who prefers conventional sexual activities.

Vixen A woman who has sex with men at the encouragement of her primary partner (usually known as a stag).

Voyeur / Voyeurism A voyeur is a person who enjoys watching others having sex, i.e., an individual who engages in voyeurism.

CONFESSION I: CANDY

After completely reinventing herself at the age of fifty-two, the only thing sweeter than Candy's name was her post-sex craving for sugary treats and her voracious appetite for significantly younger men.

Candy was on the traditional path for the first part of her life: grew up in a small town, met a boy after college, was married by her early thirties, and had two beautiful daughters. But Candy had a bisexual naughty side that she had repressed throughout most of her early life. Such behavior was not accepted in the community that she had grown up in. However, her husband welcomed Candy's bisexuality, and after moving to the Bay Area, they got involved in the San Francisco swinging scene. They quickly found that having an extra woman was what they both liked best.

Life happens though, and after over twenty years together, the marriage had run its course. Candy took stock of her situation: she was over fifty, divorced, very successful, and unwilling to get married again. She didn't need a man to support her. She tried to date, but unfortunately, it wasn't very successful as she was often left bored by the age-appropriate men she met. She gave it up after a few years, wondering if that was the end of dating for her.

Her Young Stud

Unexpectedly, she discovered she wasn't done, just as she was having the solar panels on her house cleaned. A small crew showed up, and one of the workers, a very young good-looking guy, caught her attention. She had butterflies in her stomach. As she walked by him, Candy locked eyes with the young worker. His muscular arms were hard to ignore in his tight-fitting T-shirt, and she couldn't help but wonder if he had washboard abs too. She thought to herself, *Oh, my God, I want to fuck him.* It felt like no one else was around as the fifty-two-year-old stared and smiled at the tall twenty-five-year-old. They chatted briefly, until the young man calmly and confidently took the conversation in a very different direction. He leaned in, lowered his voice and said: "I think you're really hot," and handed her a piece of paper.

Candy was dumbfounded when she looked at the note and saw his name and number. She thanked him for the compliment, and as he left, tried to collect herself. Over the next couple of days, she couldn't stop thinking about him. Even though he was so young, Candy couldn't help but be impressed by his boldness. *Fuck it. I don't care how old he is, he's fucking hot and I want him,* she decided.

Candy reached out to him the next day and he quickly asked her out to dinner. Two nights later she was in a bit of a frenzy as she got ready for the date. She had never been out with a guy that much younger than her and had no clue what to expect. She also couldn't believe how aroused she was when he picked her up in his truck.

As they sat together at dinner it was obvious how excited he was to be spending time with her. Out of curiosity, she asked him if he had ever dated an older woman before. He stated he had. When Candy asked how old he thought she was, he guessed forty or forty-one.

"I'm fifty-two," she confidently replied, but wondered if the age gap would be an issue for him.

He quickly replied that he found her even hotter because of it.

After they had finished dinner, they headed to his truck to drive home, but Candy decided she had other plans in mind.

"I think you should kiss me," she said as she moved closer to him.

He turned to face her. Wrapping his arms around her waist, he pulled her closer and they began to make out. The chemistry between them was intense. As the make-out session continued in his truck, his hand slid between her legs, and she whispered: "Let's find a hotel."

The minute they entered the room, they began to tear each other's clothes off. He picked her up in his strong arms and threw her onto the bed. Then he climbed on top of her and pressed his hard, naked body onto hers. As they started to kiss, she felt his arousal and thought, *My god he's huge.* As they continued to devour each other, she couldn't believe how passionate and patient that young guy was. It felt like they had been making out for thirty minutes, and he still hadn't tried to fuck her.

When she finally couldn't take it any longer, she grabbed his cock and guided it all the way in. As his hips made contact with hers, she felt every inch of him that was inside of her, and every muscle in his body that was on top of her. She was in heaven as they fucked for the next three hours. His stamina and energy were impressive.

After they had finished, as she lay there on the bed, she realized that was what she had been missing. That was what she had been waiting for. She had just fucked a guy half her age and God damn, it was fucking hot!

For the next several months, they rocked each other's worlds. Sometimes they booked a rental home for the weekend, sometimes it was just a night in a hotel. With her sex drive reignited and stimulated to a level she had never experienced before, Candy felt she was getting her groove back. When her cub finally decided to go back to school, and his availability significantly changed, the wild love affair ended. Candy had seen the light though: younger men were her jam. They were easy to hang out with and didn't want to possess her like the older men did. Ditching older guys and vanilla platforms for good, she switched to naughtier apps like Feeld and FetLife. Consensual, no-strings-attached sex was exactly what she was looking for.

Her Cuck

The minute Candy posted her pics online she was inundated with messages from hot young guys. Candy was having a blast hanging out with various local studs when someone from San Diego hit her up. She was surprised by the interest from someone four hundred miles away, but he seemed cool, so they started video chatting to get to know each other. She liked him, and their personalities meshed well, so after a month of talking online, he flew to Northern California for an in-person meetup.

When she first met him in the flesh, she felt an instant connection, as if it were meant to be. He also had a lot more experience in the kink world, and she was eager to learn from him. He was a cuck at heart and therefore was completely supportive of her fucking as many guys as she wanted. That was something new for her, and she loved it. A man who not only supported her wild desires but was actually turned on by them. From there they began to develop a deep cuck-hotwife relationship.

He encouraged her to push her boundaries, and with his support, that's exactly what she did. They started out in the swinger scene, meeting couples and singles in various arrangements. Then they began attending sex parties where Candy discovered she really liked getting fucked by a line of guys, one after the other, while her cuck stood by and watched; he loved seeing her being pleased by other men.

As Candy got more into the lifestyle, she started exploring her submissive side and discovered one of the hottest scenarios for her was to be treated like a "whore." She enjoyed nothing more than showing up at a stranger's hotel room and immediately dropping to her knees to suck his cock right in the doorway. It was invigorating playing the submissive whore, which was in direct contrast to who she was in her professional world. Living a double life only made it hotter.

One day she sent a naked photo to her cuck of her legs spread wide open. When he sent the photo back to her, he had edited it and wrote "whore" in the space between her ass and pussy, along with instructions: *Why not make this your first tattoo?*

Candy decided to go for it, and a few days later, she found herself spread-eagle on a table at a tattoo studio. To Candy's delight the tattoo artist replicated the image exactly. The minute he was done she snapped a pic and sent it to her cuck.

How do you like my new taint-too?

Her cuck was elated. When she started posting pics of her new 'taint-too,' her online popularity instantly skyrocketed. Enjoying the body modification and the online responses she had gotten from it, Candy also added six labia piercings and a Christina piercing (a.k.a a Venus piercing, placed on the top of the vulva, where the outer labia meet on the pubic mound).

Her Girlfriend

While having regular hookups with one specific couple, Candy started to develop a deeper friendship with the wife, Jasmine. Being right around the same age, the two older MILFs had a lot in common—especially their colossal craving for younger men.

It was refreshing to find another woman who understood her hypersexual attitude while in her fifties and they fed off each other's intense sexual appetite. At first, their hookups between the two sets of partners were just fun nights of vanilla swapping sex. But soon they started trying all different types of configurations for each other's bodies. Candy would ride Jasmine's strap-on while Jasmine lay on her back with her head over the edge of the bed and had her mouth stuffed with both guy's cocks. Sometimes one woman would be forced to only masturbate while she watched the other get railed by both men. Another evening Candy lay on top of Jasmine with their asses stacked in the air as one guy alternated between them. They were having fun and the sexual freedom they felt with each other was intoxicating.

Candy also loved Jasmine's taste in men: a killer body, with a beautiful cock, and mind-blowing stamina, and she always seemed to have a good one around. It meant that when hanging out with Jasmine, Candy never knew when a hot evening was going to happen out of nowhere. One night, they were just hanging out in the kitchen when Jasmine's boyfriend returned home. After he hugged Candy hello, he bent her over the counter, pulled her panties down, and dove his face deep into her from behind. She loved the intense forward approach! A minute prior, she was just chatting with her friend, then she was stomach down, ass up, and legs spread, getting her pussy licked from behind. He was so good that it didn't take long before she reached back and grabbed a fistful of his hair as she orgasmed.

When the show was over, Jasmine kissed her boyfriend and said how she loved smelling the scent of her friend on his lips. Seeing how aroused Jasmine was, Candy took her into the bedroom, pushed her on her back, and proceeded to give her a treatment of her own. Soon Jasmine was squirting like a firehose all over Candy's face, so much so that there were juices dripping from Candy's eyelashes. After Jasmine's eruption, her boyfriend proceeded to fuck the two of them for hours before they all passed out on the bed.

At 4 a.m., Candy was awakened by the boyfriend fucking Jasmine. Smiling, Candy rolled over and went back to sleep. A bit later, she was woken again when she felt him spread her legs. *Oh my God, here we go again!* she thought as he began to pound her for a second time. After the second round was over, she lay there holding Jasmine's hand and thought how kinky it was that both women were filled with cum as they fell asleep.

Things got especially delicious the next morning, when Candy was rummaging through the fridge looking for a snack. She noticed a can of whipped cream and decided a little food play was in order.

"Hey, why don't we eat this out of each other's asses for breakfast?" she suggested with a devilish grin as she waved the can in the air.

Jasmine enthusiastically offered to dine first. Grabbing the can, she motioned for Candy to once again bend over the counter and spread her ass. Jasmine sprayed the cream between her spread cheeks and the cold temperature made Candy giggle. Jasmine's face and Candy's ass were a mess in no time. Then they switched positions for Candy to have a taste. After they devoured each other's whip cream-covered bodies, the boyfriend fucked both of them again, sticky asses and all. The endless pounding that weekend left Candy walking awkwardly the next day.

As Candy and Jasmine continued on their epic journey of sexual adventures, they racked up tons of raunchy memories. While most gal pals shared things like makeup, shoes, or purses, Candy and Jasmine shared men and sexual experiences.

"Let's have a gang bang together," Jasmine suggested one day.

Candy loved the idea and was immediately on board. They searched through their combined pool of partners and agreed on five men to invite to the double gang bang that night. The women took turns watching every inch of each other's bodies get ravaged by the guys. But being on the bed together and holding hands while getting fucked simultaneously was the best. Candy was the first to experience the airtight seal, but Jasmine followed close behind. All in the name of keeping things fair between friends.

Among the many gang bangs they would share, the Vegas one was by far Candy's favorite. Five, hot, young Black men with huge cocks spent five hours taking turns on the older women. It was truly an unforgettable night. As sore as her ass was the next day, she felt as if she had died and gone to heaven.

Her Double Life

Recently, Candy had a great hookup while in Arizona while officiating a vanilla friend's wedding. She looked for a local playmate while there and wound up connecting with a Dom. He showed up at her hotel room with a bag full of gear and restrained her with a spreader bar and handcuffs. He proceeded to spank her and tease her with a vibrator for the next couple of hours. Her moans were muffled by the ball gag stuffed in her mouth while he completely used her like a living, breathing sex doll—and damn, she loved it. Her ass was red from all the abuse when he finally slid inside her. Just before he came, he removed her gag so he could finish in her mouth. She could not have been happier.

The next day she officiated the ceremony as if nothing had happened, and she smiled every time she felt soreness in her body. Sitting was especially uncomfortable, so she tried to stand as much as possible. The fact that nobody knew what she had been doing the night before made it all the more exciting. Doing ordinary things during the day and then being super naughty at night left her exhilarated. Candy could transform into whatever was needed—a hotwife, a whore, a business owner, living sex doll, or, as she had that weekend, a wedding officiant.

Candy genuinely liked being thought of as a sexual being. As a teenager, overtly sexual compliments made her feel dirty and weird, but she had reached a place in her life where she had no problem with the attention. She loved everything about sex: from watching people fuck, to being tangled in the middle of a bunch of naked bodies. Even though she considered herself a huge slut, she was selective about who she hooked up with, and predominantly looked for guys who were young, tall, attractive, and well-hung. But at the end of day, what excited her the most was fulfilling a younger guy's fantasy of being with an older woman, so she occasionally settled for a guy who was considered "average."

Variety was the spice of life for Candy and there was never a shortage of it thanks to her growing list of online playmates. Between Jasmine, her cuck, a handful of regulars, and posting ads when she traveled, the supply of partners was endless. She also continued to flaunt her kinkiness with several hardcore video clips on her newly created ManyVids account ranging from full-length gang bangs, to shorter clips that include toys, penetration, facials, blow jobs, creampies, and more.

Right from the get-go, Candy gained a huge following and became a minor celebrity. She began getting recognized in places like movie theaters and grocery stores. One day while at the airport she received an email that read: *I love your flip flops! I'm in line behind you at the gate.*

Looking over her shoulder, Candy saw a man waving at her. The guy, who apparently had a foot fetish, was overwhelmed to be in the presence of Candy and her lovely, exposed toes. She gave the starstruck fan a hug and joined him for a selfie, before getting on the plane. It was like being an amateur porn star and she loved the flattering attention.

At fifty-four years old, Candy was grateful to have found her sexual liberation and couldn't imagine ever being monogamous again. The biggest difference between her younger and current self was that she no longer gave a shit about what people thought. She also had no shame about what she was doing sexually. She was living out all the fantasies she had ever imagined, and she couldn't be happier. She was free for the first time in her life and planned to stay that way.

Based on episodes

650 - Candy Is a Hotwife MILF "Slut" into Younger Guys, Threesomes, Sex Clubs, and More

733 - Jasmine and Candy Have Had Gang Bangs, Threesomes, and Foursomes Together, and More!

CONFESSION II: SEAN & SAMANTHA

We all know that outward appearances can be deceiving—and that is precisely what Sean and Samantha thrived on. On the surface, Sean appeared to be the quintessential alpha male, but behind closed doors, he was secretly obsessed with getting pegged, wearing panties, and sucking cock. And, Samantha, his wife, was obsessed with it all too.

When Sean and Samantha met seventeen years ago, she was instantly attracted to his alpha male energy, rugged good looks, strong physique, and successful career. The icing on the cake was that Sean could go for hours in the bedroom. Samantha was in ecstasy. Dating turned into an engagement, and eventually, a marriage. For years they had an active and enjoyable sex life with Sean being very dominant and in-command, both in and out of the bedroom. They could never have suspected the turn that their sex life would take.

Opening Pandora's Box

It began very innocently one evening a couple years back. The two of them were home having a few drinks and getting frisky with each other. After all those years of marriage, they had started trying to spice things up a bit by introducing toys into the bedroom. With a vibrator here, and a dildo there, they were making it up as they went along. On that evening, maybe it was the drinks coupled with a yearning to push boundaries, Sean was feeling a little more adventurous than usual. With Samantha's gorgeous body spread out naked on the bed next to him, he picked up a dildo and said: "Hey, can I put this in your ass?"

Being in a playful mood herself, Samantha laughed and said the words that would change the course of their sex life forever: "Sure! But only if I can put it in your ass too!"

Sean's mind froze, but his body reacted in a way he wasn't prepared for. He instantly got hyperaroused. He had never considered doing anything like that before. But there he was, hard as a rock at the prospect. They proceeded to spend the rest of the evening playing with each other in a way that surprised them both.

After the success of that night, something awakened in Samantha, too, and she decided she wanted to push things further. She wanted to peg Sean. He was into the idea, so they went out and bought a strap-on. That was the beginning of Sean morphing into Samantha's little bitch in the bedroom.

Being at his wife's mercy was a huge departure from his daily life. By day, Sean was the breadwinner and protector of his family. His high-stress supervisor job required him to be in control and responsible, so he welcomed the transformation that took place at night in their bedroom.

Samantha was also discovering a side of herself that she never knew existed. She was getting so turned on by the thought of her masculine husband, who was the rock of their relationship, turning into her little sissy slut in the bedroom. The fact that it was a secret only she knew about made it all the more arousing. She loved it.

Sean and Samantha carried on like that for a while and eventually they started talking about pushing the boundaries even further. At first it was just playful talk. *What would it be like to have a third join them?* They talked about a guy coming in to fuck Samantha in front of Sean, as well as a woman for Sean to fuck. For Samantha, the thought of Sean being with another woman produced an intense negative emotional response, so she decided that was a boundary that she didn't want to cross. On the contrary, Sean was highly aroused at the thought of watching his wife with another man. Samantha wasn't sure she was ready for that, so to feel it out, they started watching MFM (male-female-male) threesome porn.

As they watched, Sean was totally into it. He got very aroused by the threesome, but Samantha was lukewarm on the experience—that is until one of the men in the video started jacking off the other guy to get him hard. Seeing that simple guy-on-guy hand job made Samantha crave more. She wanted one of the guys to get down on his knees and start sucking the other guy off.

"Hey, could we maybe watch some gay porn?" she asked.

Before they knew it, they were watching gay porn all the time. Sean loved how hot it got Samantha and the sex they had while watching it was out of this world. Then on one particularly hot and steamy night, with gay porn on the screen while they were fucking, Samatha whispered into Sam's ear: "I bet you wish it was you in that video."

To Samantha's astonishment, he replied: "Yes, I do."

To Sean the most important thing was pleasing his wife, the woman he was deeply in love with. Giving into her desires was the ultimate form of sexual servitude, even though he wasn't sexually attracted to men. But in actuality he didn't think they would do it, he figured it was just pillow talk.

But Pandora's box had been opened, and Samantha became obsessed with the idea of bringing another guy into the bedroom. The thought of getting to see her man in a hot guy-on-guy porn scene, up close and personal, was riveting. She wanted Sean to become her own personal porn star.

From Alpha Male to Sissy Slut

They started hunting for a bi-guy, so that Samantha could watch the men together, but with the possibility that Samantha could hook up with the new man too. They finally found one that they both agreed on and the night was set. When he showed up, initially Sean and Samantha were nervous, but something came over her after seeing the two men interact, and she started directing. She told Sean to get on his knees and suck the other guy, which he obediently did. Samantha was in heaven. Soon she had them switch, and then she got in on the action herself and sucked the other guy off. The evening finished with the man going down on Samantha to make sure she was fully satisfied. For the first time in his life, Sean was just an observer to his wife's pleasure, and he loved it.

After the guy had left and the two of them were alone, they both admitted they were a bit shocked at what had just taken place. Samantha asked how Sean felt about the whole thing.

"It was definitely a mind fuck but I would do it again," he stated.

As they continued to talk about the experience, they realized there were some lessons learned. Sean found that while he liked having a cock in his mouth, especially when he saw what it did to Samantha, he was really turned off by having a guy suck his cock. It totally killed the vibe for him. So, from that day forward, Sean found his role was to simply be of service to the other guy without any reciprocation. And while initially they thought that Samantha would be the center of attention for their trysts, Samantha found what she really wanted was for Sean to be the service slut for the two of them. From that day forward Samantha was the director of each experience and Sean became a boy toy who did her bidding.

Sean granted his wife the dominant role and all encounters from then on were arranged through Samantha. Sean never communicated or exchanged numbers with his playmates. For Sean, the process was all about respect for his wife. He wanted her to be comfortable with whomever entered their home and marriage.

Though being the dominant one was new for Samantha, she got more and more into it with every new experience. The fact that Sean was a heterosexual, alpha male who was fulfilling her wishes of forced guy-on-guy action made it all the more erotic to her. And while Samantha was clear that the thought of being with another man wasn't necessarily what she wanted, the door was always open. Over the next several months the sexy exploration was a trial-and-error experience with a learning curve. In the beginning, finding guys was difficult and sometimes they took what they could find, lowering their standards just so they could play. Admittedly, there were a few questionable selections that did not wow Sean. But he was all about pleasing his wife, so Sean dutifully went along each time in a desire to be the perfect sub for her. With practice though, Samantha got much better at vetting. They agreed it was smarter to take their time and search for the perfect match, even if it took longer to find him.

Samantha got very picky as she learned exactly who she wanted to see Sean with. Physical attractiveness was essential to her. This meant they had to be fit and muscular since Sean and Sam were gym junkies. Most importantly, suitors needed to exhibit dominant tendencies, and they had to be okay with being filmed.

Capturing the moments with videos and pictures was a big turn-on for Samantha, and it became a critical component of their hookups. Samantha wanted to build up her own personal collection with Sean as the porn star, exactly what she had fantasized about all those months prior during their very vanilla evenings of watching gay porn. So if a guy wasn't down to be on tape, it was an instant deal breaker.

Less concerned with chemistry, Sean preferred average to large cocks and considered small ones a waste of time. Above all, the true excitement for Sean was performing his servitude while his wife watched. Without her, it could not exist.

Understanding that some guys had performance anxiety fucking another man in front of his wife, Sean was occasionally allowed to play solo with the guy under one condition: they had to record the entire scene and send it to her immediately afterward.

A Cock Cage and Panties

Sean and Samantha went along like that for a while, thinking they had reached the limit of their kinky wild sides. One day, while they were in a sex shop picking up some toys for Samantha, they stumbled upon a cock cage.

"What do you think of this?" Samatha asked, holding it up for him to see.

For Sean, he saw in the cock cage a way to escalate his submissive role to an even greater level. The cage became a symbol of his service and devotion to both the man and Samantha. Sean also found that being restrained took his focus off of his own needs and reminded him that the other man's pleasure was all that mattered. It made it impossible for him to forget he was not an equal. Sean was there to dutifully suck cock and bottom with no reciprocation.

After each session, the men would leave and Sean would eat his wife's pussy and use toys on her until she felt she was fully satisfied. With his cock caged and rendered useless, chastity became a viciously tantalizing game for the couple. Not coming also kept him hornier since there was no post-orgasm exhaustion, plus the absence of penetrative sex with Samantha required them to be intimate in different ways. As a result, their emotional and mental connection grew so much deeper.

What started as an evening soon turned into a full day of cock restraint. From there it became a week. The more he was denied, the more he wanted his wife. The more he wanted his wife, the more she denied him. When he was finally allowed to orgasm after a week of denial, the release was beyond anything that he had ever experienced. The longest she had ever denied him was a month and a half. They felt that anything beyond that length ran the risk of losing the appeal. As a bonus, it created a barrier so the gay and bi guys could never get too close to Sean's genitals. Protected from unwanted advances, he could completely relax into his role as a sex slave during the sessions, and eventually, he refused to play without it.

One day while shopping, Samantha saw a cute little pair of panties and thought, *I wonder what Sean would look like wearing these.* She bought the panties, brought them home, and told Sean to wear them. He of course obliged, and when he saw how happy Samantha was when he put them on, he started to wear them all the time.

One of Samantha's favorite things was making him wear them while they were working out in the gym. She loved seeing him all sweaty, in his manly workout clothes looking tough. But secretly knowing that under all that alpha-male hotness was a pair of lacy female panties drove her wild.

Sporting them under his clothes while running errands or dining at a restaurant was another dirty little secret that bonded them. Even at home, while brushing his teeth and seeing his reflection wearing panties, stockings, or thigh-highs, helped reinforce his reality of being her loyal sub. Honestly, the only reason he could think of not to wear them was the possibility of someone accidentally seeing them. The last thing he needed was his golf buddies sneaking a peek at the pretty panties when he bent over. That would be too much to handle. But the risk was also a part of the thrill, so she demanded he always wear them.

Eventually she purchased crotchless panties for him and after he put them on, she made him bend over and stick his ass in the air as if he was getting ready to receive a pegging. He looked so degraded in them. So much so that she decided to float the idea of anal sex.

"What if instead of me pegging you like a little sissy, it's actually one of my guys with their cock up your ass?

Her wish was his desire, so onto all fours he went at the next session and took the guy's cock right up his ass. As a good sub, Sean never dared comment or critique his superior's performance and took the ass fucking like he was supposed to.

In addition to the one-night stands, Sean developed an ongoing hookup with one guy. Standing over six feet tall, the towering gay man exuded the domineering stature Samantha craved for her sub. Over time he became more than just a no-name hookup, Samantha actually liked who he was as a person. Thanks to his respectful attitude, he was granted permission to see Sean privately. He had no problem being videotaped and the way he communicated with Samantha ahead of time, got her worked up. Reading messages like, *I can't wait to fuck your husband,* or *I am going to destroy his ass tonight,* sent her over the edge. Although Samantha stepped out of the room when he arrived, the camera was constantly recording. Hearing the guy report, *I came three times last night,* made Samantha so proud of her slut.

Up until that point Sean hadn't been wearing the panties for his hookups with the men since Samantha assumed they wouldn't be into it. But for Valentine's Day, Samantha messaged their regular: *I know it's not really your thing, but would it be okay for Sean to start off wearing red crotchless panties this evening?*

She assured him that the panties could be removed right after the initial hello. But not only was the regular okay with the panties she found out he was also into them. When Samantha watched the videotape later, she laughed when she saw the regular wear them as well. That started a trend and Sean started modeling his fancy lingerie for all their dates. Sean's transformation into Samantha's personal little sissy slut was complete.

Samantha Joins In

Shortly after, Sean got a special treat when Samantha found the courage to fuck her first guy in front of him. He was a bi guy coming over for Sean, but after seeing his hot pics, she realized she was attracted to him and wanted in on the action. When she asked Sean if that would be okay, he quickly replied: "Hell yeah, I've been waiting for that!"

Getting ready thirty minutes before the date, Samantha's heart raced as she worked herself into a frenzy. She was nervous to be fully intimate with a man in front of her husband. *What was he feeling?* she wondered. *Would Sean look at me differently the next day? Was it perhaps a line we shouldn't cross?* She was nervous about screwing up the wonderful dynamic that they had. But as far as she could tell, their marriage couldn't have been going better.

Samantha also knew that their relationship had reached levels of intimacy that they never expected, and she now felt closer to Sean than she ever had. Their relationship felt so solid that she reasoned it would probably be okay even if things didn't end up as fun as they imagined. Still though, she voiced her concerns to Sean. He assured her that he really was dying to see her get fucked.

In truth though, Sean wasn't exactly sure how he would handle it. He knew he might get jealous, but he also understood that there was no reason to. He figured a little jealousy was probably a good thing as long as it did not reach an unhealthy level. *Just suck it up, buttercup,* is what he decided to tell himself, if it got to be too much. The last thing he wanted to do was ruin the experience for Samantha.

That night Sean obediently fluffed the guy for his lovely wife so that she could get properly fucked. As he was blowing the guy, all he could think about was how fucking hot it was going to be to see Samantha finally getting off properly from another man. With his cock cage on, Sean sat back and finally got to watch his wife get fucked. It was the hottest thing he ever saw, and something they decided to keep doing.

Turns out, finding guys that could fuck both of them was an immense thrill. Sharing the same cock, on the same night, during the same date, enabled them to bond to an even higher level. And comparing stories afterward led to some kinky conversations. If Samantha asked, "How did his dick feel for you?" Sean could literally ask her the same thing.

Interestingly, Sean never wavered on his sexuality, but he did question what it meant for his alpha male personality. He was sure embracing his sissy side did not negate his alpha persona, but for them to coexist, he decided that a balance needed to be maintained. Being a sub in the bedroom 24/7 was not appealing to him. When he discussed this with Samantha she completely agreed, since one of the things she loved most about him was his dominant, alpha male persona. They agreed that they would have to switch it up with some regularity so Sean could take charge in the bedroom, and fuck her like the alpha male he is. It allowed them to achieve the balance that made all the other wild and crazy bedroom antics work for them.

Sean admits that he often wonders if they should stick with what they have been doing or keep pushing limits. *Was there a gang bang in their future?* Sean began thinking about entertaining multiple men at the same time, and how many cocks could he handle as he got them ready to fuck Samantha. As long as Samantha could gather enough guys that checked off all of her boxes, the couple admitted they were both open to finding out.

But for now, they are content. Even though keeping secrets could be exhausting, Sean is grateful to have Samantha, and Samantha is grateful that she has Sean. The freedom to be vulnerable and trusting with each other was a privilege neither of them ever took for granted. They both saw how many couples in the world who did not have the same level of trust, and they felt blessed to have that in each other. A supportive partner whose love never wavered was a gift beyond compare.

Based on episodes

774 - Samantha and Her Alpha Husband Love Pegging, Guy on Guy Action, MMF 3somes, and More

780 - Sean Is an Alpha Male into Guys, Hotwifing, Cock Cages, and More

CONFESSION III: ASHLEY

Most people don't wind up having a threesome with their best friend's mom and stepdad, but Ashley wasn't most people. Her salacious story began back in high school during frequent sleepovers at her best friend's house.

The more time she spent around the family, the more she noticed that attractive couples would frequently pop in. She was intrigued by the constant parade of sexy strangers and wondered what exactly was going on. *Were the rumors she heard about them being swingers actually true?* Just the idea of it made Ashley's mischievous mind wander.

One afternoon, the friend's mother left her phone in the home office and Ashley dared her pal to get it. She didn't believe her friend was bold enough to do it, but surprisingly, the friend accepted the challenge. As they scrolled through the messages, they were shocked to discover a slew of steamy texts and naked photos from other couples, men, and women. It overwhelmingly confirmed the rumors she had heard: her best friend's parents were indeed swingers.

Ashley, being a lot more mature for her age than her friend, became close with the mom over time. They often stayed up chatting long after her friend went to sleep. One night when they were hanging out, Ashley boldly asked the mom what she thought about open marriages. The mom laughed and said she knew they had looked through her phone and explained: "After twenty years of marriage, sometimes you need a little something to keep it fresh."

Then the mom quickly shut the conversation down and made it clear the topic was off-limits. But it was something Ashley never forgot.

How it All Started

Ashley and her best friend drifted apart over time, and she lost contact with the family for many years. During that time though, she heard that her friend's parents had gotten a divorce.

Ashley was surprised when five years later the friend's mom randomly reached out to see how she was doing and let her know that she was missed. Happy to hear from her, Ashley agreed to meet the mom and one of her other daughters for lunch. During the meal, the mom invited Ashley back to their house to hang out for a bit. Ashley gladly accepted.

As the two of them sat on the couch together talking about what they both had been doing over the past five years, Ashley couldn't help but notice the mom's new husband was extremely attractive. She wondered if they were swingers, just as the mom and her previous husband were.

Young, hot, and *very* single at the time, Ashley had actually started exploring alternative relationships herself. Finding it hard to meet decent single guys, she started looking for couples. She soon began messaging with a couple who were a little bit older than her and extremely hot. After several weeks of texting, she gathered the courage and hooked up with them twice. She had her first girl-on-girl experience with them and even made the woman squirt. She had a great time and realized that she loved being a unicorn. She couldn't wait to do it again and was on a mission to have more unicorn experiences.

The next time she spoke to the mom, she decided to share her recent experience. After some idle chitchat she boldly announced:

"I recently had a threesome with a couple I met on Tinder, and it was hot as fuck!"

She then asked the mom if she and the new hubby were playing with others as well.

"Oh no, he would never allow that because he is so protective over me. He's definitely not open to it," she explained.

But she did confess that her new husband thought Ashley was attractive. As the banter escalated, Ashley saw an opportunity and decided it was time to make her move.

"I think you're actually both hot as fuck."

She then revealed that she had been lusting after the older couple since that day they had lunch together and hung out at the house. With her intentions out in the open, the three ended up low-key flirting and exchanging racy photos in a group chat. It became apparent that all three were into each other and Ashley was turned on just thinking about the fact that she was possibly going to fuck her ex-best friend's mom and stepdad.

Making a Threesome Happen

As the X-rated texting continued, her desire to fuck the couple became unbearable. Determined to make it happen, one night she hopped in her car and drove to their house. Not knowing what to expect, she was filled with a mixture of fear and arousal. Upon arrival, the mom was very excited to see her, but she noticed the husband was quiet and distant. Ashley worried she had made a huge mistake. *What if he had changed his mind about her?* With a noticeable tension in the air, Ashley asked the wife for a tour of the house. When they got to the primary bedroom, Ashley voiced her concerns and suggested postponing the potential threesome but the wife insisted it was still on.

"Oh, trust me, he is absolutely into it! He wants it just as much as you and I do," the mom assured her.

That was all Ashley needed to hear. She leaned in and boldly planted a kiss on the mom. She instantly leaned into it, grabbed Ashley's hips, and pulled her closer. Her body was a perfect ten! She was overwhelmed with excitement as her hands fondled the mom's voluptuous breasts. Touching her was pure bliss and the make out session seemed to last an eternity. Ashley couldn't believe it was really happening. Then the mom pulled away and seductively exclaimed: "Oh my God, that's hot! Now I want you to go downstairs and do that to my husband!"

As they walked downstairs, Ashley was nervous. Seducing a man she barely knew in person seemed intimidating, but she was up for the tantalizing task. Mentally psyching herself up, Ashley followed as the mom led the way.

When the two returned downstairs, the mom stepped outside for a cigarette. Noticing her watching through the blinds, Ashley took a deep breath before bravely walking over to the quiet husband. Without exchanging a single word, she crawled onto his lap, straddled him, and began kissing him. He came alive instantly and it was game on.

"I like what I'm seeing and I want to join in," the mom stated as she walked back inside.

Ashley remained straddled on the husband, turned on by the risqué situation.

"Well then take your clothes off and get in here," Ashley responded.

The mom walked over, sat down beside them, and the three of them started going at it. Soon the mom spun Ashley around on the husband's lap so she was facing outward. Then she got on her knees and proceeded to go down on Ashley as the husband fondled her breasts; it was electric. As the mom went down on her, Ashley could feel the husband's rock-hard cock through his pants and all she could think about was getting it into her mouth. Without saying a word, she got his cock back and forth between their mouths.

After playing for a while in the living room, they ended up back in the master bedroom where the oral sex continued. First, Ashley devoured the mom's pussy and then she sucked the husband's well-hung cock till he exploded in her mouth. The real pleasure came when at the mom's command, the dad pulled Ashley's legs to the edge of the bed and fucked the shit out of her. Good Lord, the husband's cock was seriously big and he knew exactly how to use it to drive her crazy. As he was fucking her, the mom slipped a finger inside Ashley's ass, taking Ashley to a place she had never been before. *What the fuck is going on? Is this really happening?* she kept thinking. She felt like she was dreaming. It was during that night that Ashley experienced her first orgasm thanks to her talented older lovers.

Exhausted after hours of hooking up, the three of them snuggled in bed with the husband in the middle. As the wife drifted off to sleep, he started rubbing Ashley's leg and whispered dirty things in her ear. Realizing his massive cock was hard again as it pressed into her thigh, Ashley got turned on. Not wanting to wake the wife who was sleeping soundly, the two of them crept downstairs.

She laid down on the couch and as he positioned himself on top of her the two of them started making out. It was one of the hottest, raunchiest, make outs she had ever had. By the time he rolled her over and fucked her from behind, she was dripping wet. The entire time he was fucking her she kept thinking about the fact that the man's wife was peacefully sleeping upstairs. It was so naughty that she quickly had her second orgasm of the night.

The next morning when they told the mom that they had fucked while she was sleeping, the three enjoyed a good laugh. Everything seemed to be perfect and from that point on, the three of them continued to hook up. Ashley relished in being their sexy unicorn and hoped the naughty fun would never end. And for a while, it didn't. She started going over to their house regularly and sometimes when the stepdad wasn't around, she would just hook up with the mom. One of Ashley's favorite things was to get on her knees under the mom's desk and go down on her while she was hard at work.

How it Ended

One day, out of the blue, the husband messaged Ashley and told her that the mom's fantasy was for him to go out with Ashley alone. It was an unusual request, but Ashley was eager for the chance to be alone with him again. She was still turned on thinking about that first night when they fucked while the mom slept upstairs.

The night of the "date," Ashley met him at a restaurant and was confused when he presented her with a beautiful bouquet of flowers. She was under the impression they were meeting for a fuck, but it seemed different. After having a very intimate dinner together, they ended up talking in his truck for over two hours. All Ashley wanted to do was to go fuck, so when he suggested they get a hotel room, she quickly agreed.

When they got to the room, Ashley could immediately tell something was different. He was taking his time, talking to her slowly, making her feel like the center of his world as he took her clothes off. The sex was hot but in a completely different way. Instead of being raw and raunchy, the sex was sensual and intimate. As much as Ashley enjoyed it, she felt that a line had been crossed.

Though Ashley was never clear if the mom was totally down for what took place between them, what was clear was that the stepdad started acting differently after that night. His communications with her became more emotional and intimate in nature.

Even though Ashley began to feel uncomfortable with the situation and didn't know if he had told the mom what happened that night, she did hook up with the two of them again. One afternoon while the couple were in her town, they invited her out for lunch.

It was after lunch when things got hot and heavy. In broad daylight, in the restaurant parking lot, they all hooked up in the front seat of the couple's truck. While Ashley sat in between them, they started taking her clothes off. Soon she was on her knees on the floorboards of the truck sucking the husband's cock while the couple made out. As he pulled her up off the floor, the mom climbed on top, and rode him until she came. Then Ashley got her turn to ride him while the wife alternated between kissing them both. Though the whole thing was over in twenty minutes; it was hot as fuck and Ashley was left as usual, wanting more.

Unfortunately, it was right after their hot threesome in the truck that things got messy. Ashley started getting texts privately from the husband. Even though she felt bad about it, she started seeing him behind the mom's back. But he fucked her so good, it was really hard to say no.

Their secret affair didn't last long. Things exploded when the mom found out she was at the house fucking the stepdad. Turns out the household security cameras were still on, and the mom had seen everything! It blew up their marriage and Ashley felt awful at the realization that she was now a certified homewrecker. Though the husband then claimed he wanted to get divorced to be with Ashley, she wasn't interested and told him so. She knew he was not to be trusted and figured he was just infatuated with her because she was young and hot. She was wise enough to know that even though they had great sex, they didn't have a genuine connection.

Although Ashley ended things with him, every so often he would text her: *Hey baby, I miss you.* Which always pissed her off.

She felt bad about what she had done to the mom and had no desire to speak to him again. Ashley moved on with her life but didn't leave her sexually adventurous ways behind. Instead, she sought out new couples to have more threesomes with because being a unicorn for couples was still hot to her.

Ashley made the most of her roaring twenties, sexually exploring as much as she could. She was having a blast and was in no way looking for commitment or to fall in love. However, when she unexpectedly met a cute lesbian at work, life took an unexpected turn. Even though she had always been physically attracted to women, Ashley never thought she would ever be in a committed relationship with anyone. But the more she connected with her coworker, the less she could deny the attraction to that woman, so she pursued her. Soon after, the flirtatious coworkers began sleeping together and very quickly fell in love. They are currently engaged and although she has settled down, Ashley will never forget the unbelievably hot times she had as a wild unicorn!

Based on episode

740 - Ashley Had Threesomes with Her Best Friend's Mom and Stepdad, and It Ended Badly

CONFESSION IV: BETTY

Betty is a soccer mom with a "mom bod." So how did she wind up as a hotwife who's into threesomes, double penetration, gang bangs, and more?

Betty was a fairly promiscuous youth, always craving an endless supply of sex. "Slutting it up" in high school, Betty maximized the potential for keeping her pussy entertained. She had a list of guys and after she had her way with one guy, she would always call another.

After getting married, like a lot of long-term couples do, Betty and her husband's monogamous sex life suffered from routine. But when Betty became pregnant with her second child, her husband became unusually aroused by the changes to her body. Hot and heavy once again, he couldn't keep his hands off her voluptuous physique. As the dirty talk increased in the bedroom, he blurted out something that even Betty was surprised by: "I'd love to see you fuck another guy."

After ten years of marriage, that honestly sounded pretty good to Betty. The couple joined a swinger's site and started checking out other couple's profiles together. Since Betty was the only woman her husband had been with sexually, she thought it was a good opportunity for him to explore as well.

They had a few soft-swapping experiences with other couples, but over time, it became apparent that her husband was not interested in fucking other women. He hardly even watched porn. He was very happy to have Betty be his one and only, and was solely interested in watching her get attention from other guys. So eventually he pushed her to do more.

"I want you to go out and get fucked by someone else. Then, I want you to come home and tell me about it," he requested.

Being a hotwife suited Betty just fine and she immediately got on the apps to start searching. As a mother of two, Betty had normal insecurities about her post-baby body—with stretch marks and a few extra pounds—but the overwhelming amount of attention she received from guys dying to fuck her made her feel like a goddess. Being so highly desired by the opposite sex allowed her to embrace her short, full figure. Plus, the fact that no guy she messaged ever failed to reply boosted her confidence even more.

Becoming a Hotwife

One day she opened one of the apps, and there he was . . . an honest-to-God bull. He was hotter than fuck and larger than life. She corresponded with him over the next few weeks, and they finally agreed to meet. As she sat in the hotel room, she couldn't believe she was about to meet her bull. Betty was nervous as she heard the knock on the door. She composed herself and took a deep breath, reminding herself that her husband was 100 percent on board with it.

Betty tried to appear calm and confident as she welcomed him into the room but he could tell she was nervous. He calmly walked over to her, put his hands on her shoulders, told her it was all going to be fine and that she could stop any time she wanted to. Before long, they were kissing, and she realized she was ready for anything. The bull's hands started roaming all over her curves, grabbing her large breasts and, pinching her nipples hard. She let out little screams of ecstasy, fully turned on by the pain and pleasure.

Then, she reached down and began rubbing the bull's cock through his jeans. He was already hard, which made her want to gag on it. She got down on her knees, unzipped his pants, and started blowing him. The intensity of sucking his cock was incredible. She devoured every beautiful inch of him, with her saliva running down her hand and arm as she worked him.

"Oh, my God, you're so fucking good with your mouth," he exclaimed.

That was absolute music to her ears. It had been so long since she heard anything like that. Finally, when she couldn't take it any longer, she got on the bed and begged him to fuck her.

Returning home after getting the "stuffing fucked out of her," she triumphantly entered the house, walked over to her husband, and kissed him as if they hadn't seen each other in a month. He grabbed her, and lifted her up on the kitchen counter, then began to go at it as Betty described in detail exactly what had gone down with the bull. Life was good.

After the success of her first experience, Betty had another, and another, and then another. Hotwifing energized Betty—she found that the more sex she had, the more sex she wanted, and as a result, would return home in desperate need of even more sex with her husband. Her husband loved her hotwifing too. Letting his mind wander as he imagined what Betty was doing each minute she was gone, was thrilling. And each time she returned home, they got off recounting the juicy details as they reclaimed each other.

Threesomes and Moresomes

With her newfound freedom, Betty became even more insatiable. After several successful solo dates, she realized there was no need to limit herself to just one guy, so she decided to try two. Something about being able to suck one guy while another fucked her from behind was exhilarating. The combination of having her mouth and pussy used simultaneously made her feel like a certified slut. But soon, Betty got bored with MFM (male-female-male) threesomes. Realizing both her hands were still technically available when her mouth and pussy were occupied, she had an epiphany.

"I need more guys, two is not enough. I want to see how many I can handle at once," she told her husband.

He was elated and suggested she try a gang bang. When Betty connected with an older man on an app who organized gang bangs, their wish was granted.

The man told Betty he loved setting up gang bangs for married women and had a large list of vetted men she could select from.

"I can supply you with a lot of cock," he told Betty.

Whatever kind of men she wanted, he could provide. She could choose body type, age, skin color, cock size, and more. He told her once she selected the participants, all she had to do was show up and have fun.

As they browsed through the portfolio of eligible bachelors, Betty cared about cock size first and foremost. Although she preferred fit, leaner bodies, she didn't concern herself with anything above the belly button. Things like eye color, hairstyle, or facial hair were irrelevant to her. Frankly, she didn't even want to be bothered by insignificant details like their names or professions. As long as they were kind, respectful, and well-hung, they would suffice. Betty and her husband were amazed at how efficient working with an organizer was. With the event officially scheduled and the guest list confirmed, Betty anxiously counted down the days until her first gang bang.

For the personalized gang bang, the organizer prepaid for the room, and showed up with a silk rose and a bottle of tequila for Betty. Free from the hassle of hosting duties, she and her husband arrived for the festivities at the designated time. Dressed in a corset that accentuated her curves and a pair of high heels, all eyes were fixated on her as she walked through the door.

After a quick wave hello to the roomful of guests, she briefly stepped into the bathroom so the men could undress. When she returned, the studs were naked and standing at attention, ready to strike.

She looked over at her husband in the corner of the room, gave him a wink, climbed onto the bed, and laid down. She couldn't believe her eyes as she scanned the scene. Four naked men were standing in front of her, slowly stroking their cocks. She could see the lust in each man's eyes as she scanned the room. She was ready to live out her gang bang fantasy, and the best part: her husband would be watching on the sidelines.

As the night continued, one man after another took on Betty. She loved how when one man came, there was another ready to take over. The smell of sex permeated the room. Her body was drenched with sweat and cum. The more they fucked her, the more she wanted. It was almost like an out-of-body experience having different men's hands, lips, and cocks all over her.

Betty loved being treated like a queen by her lustful admirers. As the star of the show, she demanded respect and praise. The more they worshiped her body, the more she offered in return. Whether they wanted to get sucked or fucked, she was game. The ability to rotate guys meant Betty was never left waiting for someone to get hard. When one needed a break, there were several more to take his place. With these sex parties lasting two to three hours, she did not quit until every guy had sufficiently gotten off.

Betty believed in the motto "the more, the merrier," so if the organizer was in the mood to play, she gladly gave him a blow job too. Some of the younger guys recovered quickly and were able to continue fucking, which always impressed her. In fact, the challenge to outlast them all was one of her favorite parts of the whole session.

Her doting husband was always present for the gang bangs. He thoughtfully curated a new playlist for each gathering and thoroughly enjoyed quietly watching her jaw-dropping performances from the corner of the room. He never participated in the action, undressed, or even jerked off, which was his preference. Instead, he was the supportive cheerleading cuck who took photos and distributed water to the exhausted men. The decision to save his pleasure for when he and Betty were alone was how he prolonged the erotic experience. Knowing how horny he must've been by the time they returned home, she always took a nice long shower before climbing into bed with him, just to torture his aching loins a little longer.

In addition to gang bangs, Betty and her husband occasionally played with guys privately. A few of the gang bang participants were so good, they were invited to fuck her at home. Of course, hosting at home had its own challenges, and juggling their fun around their family was tricky. But they found a way to make it work. When the kids spent the week visiting their grandparents, the couple made the most of an empty house. Each night, a different gentleman was scheduled to fuck her.

Betty could never have imagined she would become a full-fledged, gang bang girl. When it became a reality, she decided it was a great opportunity to push her boundaries even further. She wanted to try her first double penetration. Since anal sex was not part of her and her husband's sexual repertoire, she specifically requested the organizer provide a knowledgeable performer.

When she finally welcomed a cock in her pussy and ass at the same time, it paved the way for her to entertain at an even higher level. The more holes she could stuff, the more men she could invite. As they continued increasing the number of attendees, the most she serviced in an evening was six. Relishing in her sexual liberation, Betty's goal was to complete a dozen gang bangs.

An Affair

Unfortunately, she didn't make it as their gang bang phase fizzled out before she could finish. Sadly, life got in the way of carnal fun for various reasons. When Betty lost her job, priorities shifted, and cutting back on expenses like hotels and babysitters became essential. In addition to the burden of financial strains, her fifty-six-year-old husband's sex drive started fading, and his excitement at the wild fun disappeared. Betty was fifty and still horny, but without her husband instigating the wild play, it didn't feel right to keep going. She rationalized that they'd had a good run, and wild memories were better than nothing.

Without a sexual connection, intimacy within the marriage subsequently dwindled as well which left Betty feeling like a roommate instead of a lover. Mourning the loss of her salacious sex life, she was unexpectedly revitalized.

Betty had a platonic friendship with a male coworker, two decades her junior whom she had known for many years. Her husband was acquainted with him as well. Betty and the thirty-three-year-old had developed a close bond during the long hours they spent together at work. One day, he confided in Betty that he was having issues with his girlfriend because she wanted to explore playing with another female. At first, Betty tried to comfort him while remaining neutral and distant but eventually she took a more intimate approach.

"Sometimes opening a relationship can work. My husband and I have been open for a long time," she admitted.

Betty couldn't believe she said that sentence out loud. What was she thinking? Betty knew that if you judged her by job and appearance, no one would ever suspect she had fucked so many guys, that even she had lost count. She had never divulged her raunchy activities to anyone, not even her closest girlfriends. She didn't think they would be able to comprehend her husband pimping her out, so she kept it a secret for all the years. When she told her coworker who she really was behind closed doors, she honestly felt relieved to finally reveal the truth to someone.

He told her he wasn't surprised and always had a feeling they were swingers ever since he saw the extra room in their house that seemed suspiciously like a "boom-boom room." He admitted that since that day he saw her in a whole new light and had thought about fucking her on more than one occasion. He even jerked off while fantasizing about it. *Wow, what a compliment!* Betty thought as her pussy tingled. She couldn't believe her ears.

In their seventeen years of friendship, Betty had never thought about him sexually but after finding out about his infatuation, things instantly changed. Now, she couldn't stop envisioning him ripping off her clothes and mounting her. Once he mentioned he had broken up with his girlfriend, the sexual tension between them increased. One night, as they hugged goodbye after a long day at work, they never let go. Before she knew it, she was sitting in the passenger seat of his car, stroking him while he drove like a madman to the nearest motel.

They were barely inside the room before Betty was on her back with her legs spread, enjoying her young admirer's beautiful body on top of her. Getting fucked once again felt fabulous. After three years of no sex, Betty was on fire and had orgasm after orgasm. The experience left her satiated in a way that she hadn't been for quite some time, and she realized there was no putting the genie back in the bottle.

When she returned home, her adult children were visiting for the holidays. Betty tried to remain composed as they chatted in the living room, but the vivid memory of what she had just experienced less than an hour prior made the mundane conversation quite surreal. She knew she was glowing and all she could think about was seeing him again.

Betty and her office boy toy fucked after hours whenever the timing was right. Having a younger lover proved to be exactly what she needed. One session would finish, they would take a short break, and then he would be ready to go again. Sometimes, he even remained hard after coming and just kept going. It was magical to her. She literally wanted to see him every night but that wasn't practical.

Betty was ecstatic to be fucking again, but also torn since her husband was not aware of her activities. Years before, she would have been delighted to tell him about screwing a young virile hunk. Undoubtedly, her husband would have gotten so aroused at all the juicy details and they would have fucked long into the night. But, due to their current detached emotional status and nonexistent chemistry, Betty wasn't sure how he would respond. Although she didn't regret the act of getting laid, she worried disclosing it would do more damage than good.

It had been years since Betty and her husband had sex, so one New Year's Eve, with Betty's drive on full speed, she felt it was worth a try. Unfortunately, the experience was without passion and ended up feeling very mechanical to her. After thirty years of building a life together, she wondered if the passion with her husband would ever be rekindled. She felt guilty at how much she was craving other men, but she also found comfort in knowing they still found her irresistible. She did not want to give up that feeling.

The affair with her young lover lasted for a few more months and as it fizzled out, so did her marriage. Though she still loved her husband and had always hoped that they could revive their connection, she realized they had grown apart and they decided to end things.

After the divorce, Betty went on to the vanilla dating apps eager to start dating. She was still super horny and dying to get back into the game. After meeting a couple of guys that were kind of okay, she met a younger guy who she just clicked with. He was a swinger and got Betty back into the lifestyle, but this time they only played together. He wasn't into her playing with bulls like her husband was, but Betty was fine with that and they're still going strong to this day.

Based on episodes

385 - Betty Loves Gang Bangs, and Her Cuckold Husband Loved Them Too

596 - Gang Bang Betty Is Swinging with Her New, Much Younger Boyfriend

CONFESSION V: MISTER MAVERICK

How do most people get turned on to the lifestyle? Some hear about it from their partners, some learn about it online, and some just stumble upon it. For young Maverick, he was introduced to it in a much more salacious way: by his father's business associate.

When Maverick struck up a casual conversation with his parent's colleague, a man he had known for years, nothing seemed out of the ordinary. One afternoon as they shot some hoops, he invited Maverick to a Halloween party he was hosting. The celebration turned out to be a great time and it was at that party that Maverick noticed the man's wife was a total knockout—a blonde with great curves—exactly his type. *Wow, this guy's a lucky man*, he thought to himself.

A Bull in Training

After that night, they continued to hang out and a deeper friendship developed. A few months later, his new friend called and asked him if he could help him move and before Maverick could even reply, he paused and said: "By the way, my wife thinks you're fucking hot."

Assuming it was a total joke, Maverick brushed it off, agreed to help them move, and then quickly changed the topic. By the time moving day arrived, Maverick had completely forgotten about the comment.

When he was finally done helping them move in, the three of them relaxed in the couple's new home with some drinks.

Everything seemed normal until the wife suddenly excused herself to use the restroom and returned wearing nothing but lingerie. *What the fuck is going on?* Maverick thought to himself.

He stood motionless trying to gauge the shifting energy in the room. He tried not to stare but it was impossible to ignore her killer body. She had big, beautiful breasts, a tiny waist, and the perfect ass. The husband quickly broke the silence: "Why don't you go over and kiss Maverick," the man said to his scantily clad wife.

With that, she walked seductively over to Maverick, and boldly pressed her lips against his. He couldn't understand what was happening. As far as he knew, most guys would be enraged if another man kissed their wife, yet there was his friend *encouraging* it.

At first the kissing was awkward. Maverick was completely out of his comfort zone, in a situation he had never been in before. But as it continued, and she took his hands and placed them on her fantastic body, he began to sink into the experience. The smell of her hair and the sensation of her shapely breasts pressed against his body made him so turned on he completely forgot about the awkwardness of the situation.

As the passion grew and they fell deeper into the make out session, she started removing Maverick's clothes. The next thing he knew his friend's wife was on her knees, devouring him. He could not believe what was happening. He was in heaven as he watched his dark skin slide in and out of her white mouth, the contrast intensified by her luscious blonde hair.

Soon, he had her on the couch, his body pressed against hers while she held his hips, guiding them as he moved in and out. His friend—her husband—just watched. Each time Maverick looked at him, his friend smiled and gave him a thumbs up. It was obvious he was turned on as he sat there rubbing his hard cock. A couple of times he came over and kissed his wife while Maverick was inside her, but he never joined in on the action. Maverick's mind was blown.

Lost in his own thoughts on the long drive home, Maverick could not believe what had just taken place. The fact that he had just had hot sex with his good friend's wife was something he had never experienced before. Figuring it was a once-in-a-lifetime opportunity, he never pushed to make it happen again, and it never did.

Swingers Clubs

Soon after, Maverick relocated to the West Coast to start a new career. While there he met a man who became his business mentor, and friend. The new mentor noticed that both he and Maverick had an appetite for beautiful white women. One day while having lunch, the mentor said: "I want to take you to a place I know you will totally love," but wouldn't say more.

A few weeks later, he took Maverick with him to Las Vegas and on the drive out, he explained that they were going to a swinger's club called Red Rooster Vegas.

As Maverick got dressed in the hotel room, he was nervous and unsure of what he was getting himself into. But he was also excited and curious about what the evening had in store for him.

Entering the main door of the club was like stepping onto a porn set. Everywhere he looked, he saw another hot scene. In one direction he saw a group of five guys taking turns fucking a woman who was on all fours. In another direction he saw a group of about ten people on a huge bed all naked and squirming over each other. Some were kissing, some were sucking, and some were fucking. It was all so hard to keep track of.

As he continued to look around, the sounds of sex filled the large room: whips cracking, and people moaning and screaming with delight; it was a total sensory overload. The mentor, who evidently was quite popular there and knew everyone from the bartender to the security guard, gave his protégé a tour. Maverick loved the vibe. Everyone was so free, relaxed, and uninhibited. He was also impressed that the club seemed to welcome all types: straight, gay, lesbian, transgender. When the tour was over, Maverick needed to sit down and compose himself as it was a lot to take in all at once.

Maverick was too overwhelmed to play that night and ended up only being a voyeur. But given the number of sexy women he saw, in all kinds of compromising situations, he knew he wanted to go back. The second time they went, his vibe must have seemed different because from the moment he walked in he was being propositioned by men who wanted him for their wives. Maverick wasn't quite ready for that yet, so he just walked around the club. Not before long he spotted a sexy woman, probably fifteen years older than him, sitting at the bar on her own. Feeling confident, he went up to her and asked if she was with anyone.

"I'm here with my husband, but he's upstairs banging his girlfriend."

She told him she was trying to find her own "friend" to preoccupy her, and looked Maverick up and down. Deciding he was the perfect distraction for her, and much to Maverick's delight, she took his hand and led him to a private playroom. Like his first experience with his friend's wife, once again Maverick was dumbstruck by his situation. There he was getting his clothes ripped off by a gorgeous married woman, whom he had known for less than five minutes.

Becoming a Bull

Maverick hooked up with a few more wives that evening before heading back to his hotel to get some much needed rest. As he lay there staring at the ceiling, he realized he loved the role he was falling into. The term "Black bull" was new to him. One of the husbands had said it, and as he thought about it, he smiled. He was in his mid-twenties, and his life was starting to open up in ways he never could have expected.

Due to his outgoing personality and respectful nature Maverick effortlessly settled into his role as a bull. Clubs were a great place to meet future playmates since face-to-face encounters were more appealing to him than searching for strangers online. He became a regular at Red Rooster Vegas and was very popular thanks to his youth, stunning good looks, and incredible ability to satisfy multiple women in one evening. Sometimes when the club closed, and he was still in the mood, he would attend a swinger afterparty and fuck some more. But he wasn't all sex all the time. Some nights he played, and other times he just socialized.

As a bull, pre-planned dates with hotwives at his house, and hookups with couples at their place were preferable to him because they were naturally more intimate. One-night stands were sometimes hot, like his first hookup at the party, but Maverick preferred hookups with hotwives he had a genuine connection with. Getting to know them and developing a connection with the husband gave him a better understanding of what was going to make the night a success. He wanted to know likes and dislikes. Limits and boundaries. Favorite erotic zones, and other insider tips so he could provide the most pleasurable experience, one that was tailor-made for each woman and couple. Most of the time the husbands just sat and watched, but sometimes they joined in, which was fine with Maverick as long as he knew about it ahead of time.

Mastering His Craft

As he continued to hook up with couples and hone his skills as a bull, Maverick started to see the subtle differences between the hotwifing couples he interacted with. His vocabulary began to include words like "cuck," "stag," "vixen," and "whore." Knowing which label to use became paramount to his success. Every couple was unique, and he realized his success depended on his awareness and flexibility to adapt to a variety of different situations. Maverick preferred a slow build process, taking time to create a rapport with the couple first. Not only did this enhance his ability to provide a great experience, but it also increased his arousal and enjoyment of the evening. He truly valued the connections.

In his dating life, Maverick bounced back and forth between vanilla and lifestyle apps. He was hesitant to reveal his swinger side when the relationships were new, or if he sensed the vibe wasn't right. He would open up only if and when the relationship became serious. After doing so, if the woman expressed curiosity, he gladly brought them to events and introduced them to the lifestyle with no pressure or expectations.

One night, Maverick brought a female friend to the club to people watch and not necessarily play. While they waited in line to enter the party, Maverick momentarily stepped away to use the restroom. When he returned, he found his date chatting with an incredibly hot Venezuelan woman. *Nice, she seems to be relaxing into the vibe,* he thought.

Throughout the rest of the evening, he noticed the hot woman constantly staring at them, and eventually they ended up chatting with her and her husband at the bar. The woman eventually asked if they wanted to play, and after checking with his date, Maverick led them to a private room.

Once inside, the other man sat in the corner to watch. Apparently, he had no interest in swapping or even playing with his own wife. Maverick turned his attention back to the two women who had stripped naked, climbed onto the bed, and had started lightly touching each other. He didn't want to interfere since he knew it was the first time his date had ever played with another woman.

He patiently waited as he watched them start to kiss. Then their hands explored each other's bodies. Slowly his date's fingers slipped inside the Venezuelan woman. As she moaned, she laid down on her back, spread her legs, and invited his date to taste her. Knowing that this was the first time she had ever gone down on a woman drove Maverick wild. He was so hard he could barely control himself, but still he waited to be invited in.

Thankfully, it didn't take much longer before the other woman beckoned him over. She hastily unbuckled his belt and lowered his pants. Maverick was in heaven as the Venezuelan goddess slid him into her mouth, as his date was still busy between the Venezuelan's thighs. When they were done with each other, the ladies laid Maverick down and as his date rode his face, the Venezuelan continued to blow him. The women switched back and forth several times, each taking their turn pleasuring him and being pleasured by him.

Maverick was happy to have the two women to himself, but he couldn't understand how the husband could just sit there and watch. He continually glanced over to the husband to make sure he was cool with it all, and each time he looked, the husband seemed happy and content to just sit in the corner and stroke himself. As long as he seemed content, Maverick was happy to continue playing with the two hot women. Even though Maverick didn't fuck either one of them that evening, the night of pure oral play was fantastic for both Maverick and his date.

Not long after that party, the Venezuelan woman reached out to Maverick to invite him over to their house to spend the night. Maverick was excited because he had been hoping to see her again. Not only because that first night was so fun and he felt a connection with her, but also because he didn't get the chance to fuck her.

In the privacy of the couple's home, the night was drastically different. Instead of sitting in the corner, the husband participated, and they had a hot threesome. The men first took turns fucking the wife. Then with her on all fours, they alternated between being in her mouth and being behind her. It was a wild and fun night for all.

Hotwife Ember Rae

Nearly all of Maverick's hookups were initiated at the club, but one of his favorite partners was found through a social media group for sex-positive content creators. The hotwife content creator, Ember Rae, was drawn to his posts that included an array of photos displaying his dominant streak. She told him she was completely aroused by the images of him blindfolding, paddling, hogtying, and gagging women. Besides being a bull, while in the lifestyle, Maverick had honed his skills as a Dom. As they continued their online connection, Ember told him that her husband couldn't abuse her in such ways because he loved her too much; he couldn't do anything demeaning to her, even if she wanted him to. Maverick, though, had no problem taking charge of her in the way she desired.

In a style true to who Maverick is, he first formed an online connection with Ember and her husband before agreeing to meet with her. When they finally did connect, they filmed the entire session so that Ember's husband could watch it later. That apparently was par for the course. Ember hooked up, filmed it, and then watched it with her husband later as foreplay for their own sexual adventures. Maverick loved being the catalyst in their relationship and even had an open dialogue with her husband for constructive feedback. Did he like the latest video they sent him? Was there anything else he wanted to see next time? Did he like the way Maverick had been fucking her? Depending on the answers, Maverick adjusted the future content accordingly. The husband was ecstatic about the way Maverick pleased his wife and Ember adored Maverick's body, especially his cock.

Maverick and Ember's connection evolved quickly to the point where she was allowed to spend entire weekends at his house. That was what Maverick loved best: the chance to enjoy quality time with a hotwife outside of the bedroom allowed him to build a deeper connection with her. He had heard lifestyle horror stories about jealous husbands, broken relationships, and even divorces, but never experienced it firsthand. On the contrary, all of his encounters were pleasant and rewarding. That was probably a testament to who Maverick was as a lover and as a person. To this day, Ember and Maverick have an ongoing connection that they both value with no plans to change it any time soon.

Over the years, Maverick learned that most husbands shared their wives because they were their favorite porn stars, and nothing beats watching live porn. Although he respects their kinks, he doesn't identify with them. Ironically, the man who made a hobby out of fucking wives admits he wouldn't be comfortable letting another man fuck his. He's not sure if it's because of the way he was raised in the South, or just a personal insecurity that results in him seeing it as a weakness. Either way, he's just not ready to cross that boundary yet. Fortunately, most of the women he dates seem to be more interested in other women than other men. He often wonders if they're being truthful, or if they are simply too shy to admit their true desires. Regardless, being with a woman who only enjoys playing with other women is currently what works for him.

A decade later, the thirty-two-year-old is still reaping the benefits of the lifestyle, not only personally but professionally. He is currently a very successful content creator and goes by the alias Mister Maverick on all platforms. He no longer frequents Vegas clubs because he prefers to stick with his carefully selected inner circle of sexy friends. Between rendezvous with long-term lovers like Ember, regular couples that he hooks up with, and the occasional holiday-themed house party, his calendar remains sufficiently booked. Though most people would consider Maverick a very successful "bull," he just considers himself "a very lucky man."

Based on episode

862 - Mister Maverick Has Been in the Lifestyle Since His Early Twenties

You can find him here: allmylinks.com/mistermaverik1

CONFESSION VI: EMBER RAE

To the outside world, Ember Rae appeared to be the typical cheating military wife. While her husband was deployed overseas, Ember slept with tons of guys. But what nobody knew was that not only did her husband know she was sleeping with other guys, he was the one who *encouraged* it.

After meeting in 2005, and marrying in 2008, the couple has been together for nearly twenty years. From the start, Ember's husband was aware of her bisexuality and didn't mind her exploring with other women.

When they moved to Virginia to accommodate her husband's military career, they discovered a salacious fact about their newest friends. The other couple confessed they were swingers and had no shame spilling the juicy details about their steamy swapping escapades. Their friends' stories about swapping partners were interesting but didn't necessarily appeal to them since Ember was not comfortable sharing her husband with another woman. However, after learning about the adult dating site the swingers used, they saw the potential to find bisexual playmates for Ember. The couple went on a few successful dates which ended with Ember hooking up with a woman while her husband watched. He knew how much she truly adored eating pussy, and while it was fun to watch her go down on a girl, he soon craved something different.

During his fourth deployment, her husband proposed an outrageously wild idea. He nonchalantly asked if she would be willing to film herself with another man. Ember was slightly offended by the request. To her, that would be the epitome of a cliché cheating military spouse.

"You must be crazy if you think I'd disrespect our marriage like that," she responded.

Her husband genuinely appreciated her loyalty but explained that he was not asking her to cheat. Since it was his idea, it was a completely different situation. It sort of made sense to her, but she still wasn't comfortable with it. She said she needed time to think about it and, in the meantime, hoped he would forget and drop the subject.

While still deployed a few months later, when his birthday rolled around, Ember realized he hadn't forgotten. On the contrary, the casual question had become a serious desire. During a phone call she asked him what he wanted for his special day, and she was not prepared for his answer.

"I want you to fuck a guy for me."

Apparently, not only did he want her to fuck another guy, he wanted her to record it so he could then watch it for his own enjoyment. She could tell by the tone of his voice he was dead serious, but it still took her a bit of time to get her warmed up to the idea. By the time they hung up the phone, she said she couldn't promise it would happen, but she would at least try.

After the call ended, Ember logged onto the adult website and switched their profile from "seeking couples" to "seeking men." It didn't take long to find exactly what she was looking for. Ember connected with a super innocent looking teacher. Aside from his dashing appearance, she was drawn to his profile which stated he had experience in the lifestyle, familiarity dealing with couples, and most importantly, he had endorsements from women he had previously played with.

At first, Ember was insanely nervous about arranging a date with a complete stranger. *What the hell's wrong with me? What if*

I get murdered in a seedy hotel room by a random stranger from the internet? she worried. As she continued to message back and forth with the teacher, her anxiousness subsided, and they set a plan in motion.

First-Time Hotwife

They met at a hotel during his lunch break, which added to the naughtiness factor. Since safety was still a legitimate concern, as planned, Ember FaceTimed her husband. Waiting in the room for the mystery man to arrive was especially nerve-racking, since Ember considered her husband her one and only. Together since they were fourteen years old, all she knew was her husband's body. Technically, she was more comfortable with female partners so the concept of touching another man was foreign to her. She instantly felt awkward and inexperienced when she heard the knock on the door.

She told her husband that she was freaking out and didn't know what to do. He suggested she start by answering the door. She hastily fixed her hair, blotted her lipstick, and glanced at her silhouette in the mirror. Then there was another knock which startled her. Ember was so frantic, that she almost forgot to press "record" on the tablet she brought to film the session. Exhaling deeply, she slowly opened the door and welcomed the handsome teacher inside.

Looking at her phone, she asked her husband what to do next and before he could answer, the teacher politely interjected.

"Why don't you come closer to me?"

Following his lead, she blew her husband a kiss via the screen and walked toward her date. Her body tingled as he ran his fingers across her arm. As he leaned in to kiss her, she closed her eyes and let the natural chemistry take over. His breath on her neck sent chills down her spine, causing goosebumps. Piece by piece, her clothes came off. Soon she was completely naked, wrapped in the arms of a new lover as her virtual voyeur husband eagerly watched.

As the teacher fucked her in various positions, she periodically glanced over to gauge her husband's reaction. Each time she looked at him, all of her worries instantly faded after seeing the enormous grin plastered across his face. When the teacher pulled out and told her to lick her juices off him, her husband's jaw dropped. Ember's oral skills were so phenomenal that the teacher's legs were twitching. Occasionally, her eyes darted to the phone screen so she could make eye contact with her husband while she serviced the other man. It was impossible to tell whose cock was harder—the teacher's or her husband's. After a few more minutes of passionately blowing him, the teacher came all over her spectacular tits. The epic finale rendered her husband speechless.

The virtual experience was much smoother and enjoyable than Ember could have anticipated. Her husband was beaming as he repeatedly thanked her. It was exactly what he had wished for, and looking in from the outside, seeing her get fucked was totally different and incredibly fucking hot.

The kinky arrangement quickly became a favorite of her husband's—and surprisingly, Ember's too. The erotic little game was the perfect way for them to stay connected while they were temporarily long-distance. Ember became quite comfortable in front of the camera and was talented at capturing the perfect angles. She found that she truly did love being on film for him. As a stag and vixen hotwife couple, there was never an element of humiliation or denial toward her husband. He simply loved sharing her and witnessing her erotic pleasure from the other men and women she hooked up with.

BBC

While he was deployed, Ember hooked up with the teacher a few more times as well as some other men. She was honestly shocked at how easy fucking other guys had become for her. With her confidence high, she was about to receive another unexpected request from her mischievous husband. One day, he randomly asked if she would ever fuck a Black man. *Whoa, where did that come from?* she wondered.

Her husband knew how much she loved having her pussy stretched and filled. He was aware of the collection of sex toys in her drawer including a pussy pump, assorted vibrators, and several giant black jelly dildos. He explained that maybe it was time she had it filled and stretched by a nicely hung Black man instead of a toy. Ember was flustered but he insisted it was time for her to find and fuck a real BBC, not a rubber one. She agreed to it and adjusted her searches to include Black men.

Back online, she was quickly drawn to a Black gentleman who turned out to be old enough to be her father. During the introductory messages, he told her he was forty-five years old. But when they met in person, she found out he was a decade older than that.

Sitting at the hotel bar together, the older man admitted he felt bad about lying, but he really wanted to meet her and was afraid his age would scare her away. Ember felt it was kind of fucked up, but she appreciated his honesty. Plus, after having seen the pictures of his enormous cock, she wanted to feel it for herself. After she decided the thirty-year age gap was not an issue, they left the bar and headed to the room. The mind-blowing sex had Ember a true believer in the saying "Once you go Black, you never go back." She gasped as his massive cock reached depths she had never experienced before. Her toes curled and her fingers gripped the sheets each time all eight inches disappeared inside her.

From then on, even after her husband came back from deployment, Ember exclusively pursued Black men. She found them extremely respectful of her marriage and invested in her pleasure. Not to mention, she absolutely loved the way their enormous cocks stuffed her tight little pussy. Even after being pounded for four hours, instead of being completely exhausted, Ember was invigorated and couldn't drive home fast enough. When she pulled into the driveway all she could think was *I can't wait to get upstairs and fuck my husband's brains out.*

Returning home after an epic night of hotwifing to enjoy the passionate reclaiming process was wonderful for her and her husband. The sex always felt completely different. Nothing could imitate or replace the high she got from being shared with another man and then reclaimed by her husband.

On those nights, her husband got to see a different, wilder side of Ember. Not to say that sex with her husband wasn't already satisfying, but reclaiming sex took it to another level entirely. Hotwifing was genuinely something they both equally relished.

To Ember, adding another person was the equivalent of using props and toys in the bedroom. It was simply another form of spicing things up, and if the arrangement ended tomorrow, Ember was sure their marital sex life would remain unfazed. But until that day comes, they were certainly going to have a good time exploring!

Random Bulls

Although hookups required trust, all partners had to undergo an extensive screening process before meeting Ember. From relationship statuses to recent STD test results, the couple tried to ensure safety was a priority. While it was easy to follow protocols when handpicking men from the swinger site, the occasional slutty night out required them to bend the rules. When Ember wanted to go out to a karaoke night at a local bar, her husband encouraged her to find someone to go home with that night, a total departure from their normal routine.

While attending the karaoke nights, Ember started to develop connections with some of the regular patrons. After a few cocktails, Ember's loose lips would secretly reveal her hotwife dynamic to guys she found irresistible. With her wedding band prominently displayed on her finger, she noticed some judgmental stares in response to her unusually flirtatious behavior. Ember chose to set the record straight before false rumors regarding her marriage spread. She told them not to worry because her husband knew what she was doing, and then told them to mind their own business.

Unlike actual lifestyle dates that progressed quickly, Ember took her time with fellow bar-goers. It was not unusual for her to be getting railed by a vetted lifestyle date within hours of exchanging the first email. However, the bar flirting organically escalated over months before resulting in sex. The most important thing was to make sure vanilla suitors who were in the friend group understood her marriage dynamic. With people in the lifestyle, etiquette and rules were common knowledge, but for outsiders, it could be confusing. Therefore, she always made it clear that fucking her would qualify as NSA (No Strings Attached) sex with zero possibility of emotional involvement.

One karaoke participant in particular became a favorite regular bull of hers due to his long thick cock, dynamite skills, and reliability. Whenever they linked up, she was guaranteed to get a good, hard fucking. Owning her nontraditional relationship choices gave Ember a sense of freedom she never expected.

Ember considered her sluttiest adventure the time she traveled to Spain with a girlfriend. While abroad, her husband wanted her to try to meet someone to film with. He figured since she was there without him it wouldn't be hard to find someone hot who spoke English and wanted to fuck her. Ironically, Ember found a man on Instagram who was also traveling.

First, she asked if the IG hottie was in a relationship. Once he replied that he was single, she explained that she was in Spain by herself and trying to find a man to shoot some sexy content with for her husband. They talked for nearly two hours, with Ember further describing the intricacies of her hotwife relationship. When the conversation ended, he drove to her hotel room and fucked her just two doors down from her unsuspecting friend. Ember tried to keep her moans and screams to a minimum as he plowed her. Knowing her friend could call or stop by at any moment while she, still married, was banging a man she just met made Ember feel extra naughty. Years later, she confessed the hookup to her friend, and they shared a great laugh over the absurdity.

Going Public

Surprisingly, Ember's husband had never been present for a live show since he was not a fan of staying out late. "Just film it for me," were his famous words. Ember Rae went on dates sometimes once a month and other times she arranged weekly rendezvous with a bull. It was much easier for Ember to get dolled up and hit the town solo than to coordinate going out as a couple. The thought of them both leaving their kids for a playdate seemed overwhelming. After all, what if there was an emergency? Eventually, one day, Ember believed they would venture out together.

Occasionally, they also revisited the topic of altering their dynamic. Ember asked if he was going to resent her down the line because of all the cock she was getting, while he wasn't getting any extra pussy. Her husband always replied that he was content.

Seeing her get fucked brought him so much joy that he didn't desire any other women. Even with his assurance, Ember still debated whether they would ever transition to a swapping couple.

Part of her was a little curious to watch her husband fuck another woman, but at the same time, she wasn't sure she could handle it. For her husband, compersion came naturally, but for Ember, it was a foreign concept. He swore he was happy and told her not to feel guilty. Having her as his favorite porn star was enough, and he urged her never to feel guilty since it was he who proposed sharing her.

One day, when she stumbled upon her stripper friend's raunchy NSFW (not safe for work) Twitter account, Ember had an epiphany. As she scrolled through the endless feed of nude photos and pornographic clips, she thought to herself, *What the fuck? I can do this*! With a massive collection of hot sex videos already stashed on her phone, she hoped to become a contender in the amateur adult content creator realm. Her only concern was if her girlfriends found out. She worried about the embarrassment.

But after some thought, she found the confidence to pursue it. She realized she didn't care if people found out. Why had she ever cared? The only person's opinion that mattered to her was her husband's and he was clearly on board. His motto was: "Fuck them, fuck everyone."

It was true that many people feared that publicly embracing their sexuality would lead to the loss of friendships, and the destruction of their reputation, or even professional disgrace. Ember, however, was in a different situation due to a chain of unfortunate events. After she graduated college with a Bachelor of Science and Pre-Law degree, three family members, including her mother, passed away within a short period of time. Emotionally taxed, her dreams of pursuing a career as a prosecutor or joining the police force were halted. As a stay-at-home mom, Ember found happiness in establishing herself as a private editor for photographers worldwide. Sadly, when the family relocated to Italy for her husband's new station, a law prohibiting military wives from working outside the base forced her to close her growing business.

Living in Italy, without a network of friends and no ability to work, she had a lot of time on her hands. Unfortunately, she couldn't open an OnlyFans page because Italy had it blocked. So instead, she decided to build her brand on Twitter and Pornhub, quickly becoming popular, and gaining a lot of fans.

When her husband was relocated back to the states, she launched an OnlyFans account with an already huge fan base. Not only did her platforms start paying the bills, but both she and her husband enjoyed the thrill of knowing that countless men were watching and experiencing her in ways she had never imagined.

Today, Ember continues to combine her hotwifing with content creating, and thoroughly enjoys herself. Seven years after beginning their hotwife journey, thirty-two-year-old Ember and her husband show no signs of stopping. On the contrary, they plan to take things up a notch. In the future, Ember is hoping to graduate from one-on-one dates to entertaining multiple men. Also on Ember's bucket list, is to be the center of attention in the middle of a gang bang. Her ideal situation would include five men—a cock for each hand and each hole would be pure bliss for her.

Based on episode

539 - Ember Rae Is a Hotwife into BBC

You can find her here: https://linktr.ee/xxemberraexx

CONFESSION VII: ROBERT

How does a completely straight man wind up wearing panties while being dominated by a man in a swinger's basement?

Robert had always been open-minded, but even he was surprised by what occurred after he bought his college girlfriend a pair of panties for their three-month anniversary. One afternoon, while shopping at a lingerie store, Robert spotted a pair of hot pink panties. He thought they were gorgeous and immediately envisioned his girlfriend wearing them. But when he proudly presented Katie with the gift, it was obvious she didn't like them. She apologized for her lack of excitement and to lighten the mood, she joked: "If you like them so much, why don't you wear them?"

"Maybe I will!" he sarcastically exclaimed as he picked them up.

Staring his girlfriend dead in the eyes, Robert performed his best interpretation of a burlesque dancer seductively getting undressed. He untied his sneakers, unbuckled his pants, and dramatically dropped them. His hips swiveled as he methodically slid the panties up his legs and then neatly tucked his cock and balls into the tiny fabric.

Framing his crotch with animated jazz hands, he shouted "Ta-da!" which made her laugh. He commented on how the material felt cool and smooth on his balls and suddenly, the ridiculous charade was not so silly.

"Don't move," Katie ordered as a serious expression washed over her face.

She rummaged through her drawers and arranged a plethora of lingerie on the bed for him to try on next.

Becoming a Cross-dresser

Robert was a petite man, so not only did everything fit him well, but the bras and panties also looked great on his slender frame. Robert and Katie both got so turned on, they couldn't keep their hands off each other. Rock-hard and ready to go, Robert pulled his cock out, bent Katie over the edge of the bed, and fucked her doggy-style. As he was about to come, Robert abruptly pulled out and flipped onto his back causing him to come all over the lingerie. Still breathing hard from the energetic session, the two of them just looked at the sticky white drops all over the lacy fabric and started to giggle. They couldn't believe what had just happened, but they continued to play dress up for the rest of the school year.

The following summer, they booked a trip to Las Vegas to visit a boutique that specializes in transforming men into women. Robert was a bit nervous, but the woman who ran the place was a gracious host and put him at ease during the entire process. The session began with a consultation where he was provided with albums showcasing different hairstyles and makeup selections. Robert opted for a more natural look to avoid looking like a drag queen. That was followed by a makeover during which Robert shaved his entire body, had his face masterfully painted, and was adorned with a shoulder-length auburn wig with sweeping bangs. Next, Robert changed into a black and white polka dot knee-length skirt and white blouse that Katie had brought.

When Robert emerged from the changing room and stood before the full-length mirror, he was shocked at how passable he looked. His reflection was unrecognizable to both him and Katie, and they decided to take a stroll on the strip. It was exhilarating to walk around outside in public as a woman, and thanks to the boutique owner's exceptional skills, no one stared or mocked him.

As they continued to walk around, the two of them got really turned on and the moment they got back into the hotel room, Katie jumped him. She pushed Robert back against the wall, got down on her knees and pulled his panties down while he lifted his skirt. She swallowed him over and over again while she ran her hands up and down his smooth legs. Then Katie told him to fuck her on the bed so they could watch themselves in the mirror. Seeing Katie on all fours as Robert, dressed as a woman, moved in and out of her, made them both come within minutes.

Afterward, while lying on the bed together, Robert realized that what turned him on was seeing himself dressed as a woman and it was at that moment that Robert identified himself as a cross-dresser.

After college, Robert and Katie split up for unrelated reasons.

Professional Dommes and Dating Apps

A few years later, Robert began seeing professional female Dommes to fulfill his cross-dressing desires. There was a dungeon located not too far from his residence, where clients could walk in without an appointment. He liked being able to satisfy his urges when they struck. It was there that Robert pursued his passion for feminization as well as humiliation. He enjoyed wearing feminine costumes such as slutty maid outfits and also living out CFNM (clothed female nude male) scenarios. It was where Robert met a Domme named Mistress Rebecca, whom he played with for two years. She was a tall, blonde Russian woman with a heavy accent and sharp features. They became close friends and sometimes Robert paid for sessions and other times exchanged household favors, like vacuuming and grocery shopping, as payment.

Mistress Rebecca excelled at pushing his limits. She encouraged him to be honest about his fetishes and provided a safe place for him to unwind. To humiliate Robert, she once had him dress up in a short red spandex dress and black patent leather heels and escorted him down the hall to another room. As he passed through the main foyer where the male security guard and receptionist were stationed, Robert kept his eyes glued to the floor. It was embarrassing for Robert to be seen by other men while dressed in women's clothing. Robert knew that they were probably used to seeing all sorts of crazy shit at their job, but he still felt humiliated and vulnerable . . . and that turned him on.

In addition to frequenting dungeons, Robert signed up for a fetish website called FetLife and uploaded a few anonymous pictures of himself wearing lingerie. He was quickly inundated with endless dick pics and vulgar pick-up lines from gay men, but he wasn't interested. Robert identified as straight and had joined the site looking for women and women only.

But, for some reason, still unknown to him, he one day felt compelled to answer a message from a man. It was short and sweet: *Those are really cute panties*

Robert politely responded: *thank you*. The sender replied and asked if Robert had any more pics of him in lingerie that he could see. *How strange to be conversing with a man about these private things,* Robert thought. But he continued to chat with him.

The man suggested Robert give him a call because texting was tiring. Robert ignored the message at first but later that evening, as he lay awake in bed with nothing else to do, he picked up his phone and called. They talked about everyday topics like sports and the weather, without discussing anything sexual.

Within seconds of hanging up, Robert received a text from the man stating he'd love to talk again sometime. Robert went to sleep without responding. The guy continued to call him over the next couple of days until Robert finally gave in and answered. Only then did the conversation slowly turn more intimate.

The man shared that he and his wife were swingers and sometimes hosted parties at their house. He told Robert he was into BDSM and although his wife wasn't, she allowed him to explore his fetish with others. He explained that although his wife was bisexual, he identified as straight, which was reassuring for Robert since he had zero interest in being with a guy.

The moment they hung up, Robert received a surprising message from the man: *Want to come over and check out my dungeon?*

Shocked, Robert demanded that the man explain his motives since he had claimed he was straight. The man simply stated that after reading Robert's profile, it was obvious they had similar kinks and he thought they could have some fun together. Then he added: *Saturday at 7 p.m. would be perfect.*

As usual, Robert refused to humor him with a response. Hours later the guy confidently sent him another message: *I'll leave Saturday open for you, just in case.*

Robert didn't understand why the man couldn't take the hint. With no acknowledgement from Robert, the pushy questions continued into the next morning: *So, are you coming over tomorrow night?*

Robert had quite enough. He aggressively typed: *NO THANK YOU,* but before he could press send, his finger paused. Suddenly, he changed his mind and erased it. And then, as if possessed by someone else, his fingers typed the words: *Is seven still good?*

The man confirmed the time and sent his address.

Robert told himself he didn't care where the man lived because he was not going. He was just being polite and would 100 percent be flaking. Early Saturday morning, Robert awoke to a new message telling him to go out and buy new lingerie, preferably white, to prove he was serious. Robert was taken aback by the balls on that guy. While still swearing that he wasn't going to go to the guy's house, he threw on sweatpants and drove to the mall.

As he perused the lingerie displays for something white, he repeatedly told himself that he would cancel the date after he found just the right outfit. He selected a beautiful matching ensemble—bright white lace panties with a garter belt and a sheer, white corset. *Maybe I should send a pic when I break the date to be nice,* he thought as he purchased the new lingerie. As he drove back home, the sentiment switched to: *maybe I'll let him see it in person for a few seconds and then I'll leave.* Then it morphed into *I hope he likes it,* as Robert put on the outfit and examined his reflection in the mirror.

As 7 p.m. neared, the man texted Robert, instructing him to park around the corner and walk to the house. He noted that the front door would be open and that the basement door was to the left. He told Robert to go down, change into the new outfit, and wait for him. Annoyed by the man's demands, Robert couldn't help but feel frustrated. *Fuck that. When I arrive, I'll knock on the door and have a serious talk with this guy and then I'll leave,* he assured himself.

As Robert drove over that evening his brain was on fire. *This is the craziest fucking thing I've ever done. I should turn around,* he thought. But as he approached the house, a powerful force overwhelmed him, and he found himself obeying the very instructions he had vowed to refuse. He walked in the front door, went down to the basement, unbuttoned his pants, and let them fall to the floor. *Fuck it. I'll just go for it and see what happens,* he reluctantly decided as he slipped into his new lingerie.

The Dom

The man emerged from the dark staircase. He was six one, fit with broad shoulders, and a stern expression. He whispered into Robert's ear that he was glad he made it. Robert, who was intimidated by the man's demeanor and stature, mumbled an uneasy "okay."

"Okay, *Sir*," the Dom corrected.

"Okay, Sir," Robert replied in a hypnotic trance.

The Dom playfully grabbed the front of his panties which caused Robert to flinch, and asked if Robert was nervous. Robert remained silent as his cock inexplicably stiffened.

"You don't seem nervous," the observant Dom noted as his knuckles pressed against Robert's semierection.

He released the waistband with enough force to make it snap against Robert's skin. The Dom escorted Robert across the room to a fancy chair adorned with leather cushions and metal studs. Several hooks with ropes hanging from them were neatly arranged on the wall behind it. The Dom expertly tied Robert's hands to the back of the chair. The ropes were tight enough to keep him from moving but loose enough not to cut off his circulation or hurt his wrists. It was obvious that the Dom was very skilled and knowledgeable in the art of Shibari.

Next, he blindfolded him.

"Are you nervous now?" the Dom asked in a condescending sarcastic tone.

Then, he pushed Robert's lips apart with his thumb and inserted his soft dick. Robert automatically swirled his tongue around his flaccid cock to explore which prompted the Dom to hastily remove it.

"Oh, you are a natural! You'll be begging for that cock by the end of the night, trust me!" the Dom chuckled.

A few moments later, Robert felt his nipples immediately harden as ice cubes were rubbed on them. The Dom grabbed one nipple and then the other and tugged on them. Robert winced in pain as each nipple was placed in a tiny, metal vice.

The Dom then tortured Robert with a vibrator, letting it linger on his dick long enough to receive pleasure, but not long enough to orgasm. The sensation was so intense it left Robert panting and gasping. Eventually the Dom, bored with orgasm control, unstrapped Robert from the chair, bent him over, and spanked his bare ass with his open palm. At first the whacks were gentle but they increased in severity over time. Robert's tolerance was further tested as the Dom traded his hand for a wooden paddle.

When he was done, he patted down Robert's swollen cheeks with a cool cloth. Robert was then positioned on a massage table with his head at the edge. The Dom ran his fingers across Robert's body wearing a textured leather glove that felt delicate and pleasurable one way, but painful the other. When The Dom's half-hard dick bumped into Robert's face, he opened his mouth, frantically searching for it with his tongue.

"You have to beg for it," the Dom reminded him.

"Please come closer," Robert pleaded so he could reach it.

"Louder! LOUDER, like you mean it!" the Dom ordered like a drill sergeant.

"PLEASE SIR CAN I SUCK YOUR COCK?!" Robert screamed.

Robert awaited his reward but he never received it. Instead, the Dom abruptly removed the blindfold and untied him. Robert was confused by the sudden ending of the session. *What the fuck just happened?* he thought, desperately trying to make sense of it all.

"Do you want some water?" the Dom asked as he sat on the loveseat across from Robert.

As he sipped his water, Robert's mind was spiraling. He wanted more. He wanted his cock. *It's now or never. What do I have to lose?* Robert thought to himself as he confidently stood up, marched over, spread the Dom's legs apart, and sucked his beautiful cock. It was the first full blow job he had ever given so he let his instincts guide him.

"I'm going to come," the Dom announced right before he pulled his cock out and came all over Robert's face.

"You did a good job," the Dom said as he patted him on the head.

"You are to leave my cum on your face until instructed otherwise. Let's go upstairs and have a beer." Covered in come, Robert followed him upstairs, carrying his clothing and backpack.

"Hello," said a female voice from the kitchen. Robert turned and was mortified to see the Dom's wife.

"Well, I guess you got what you were begging for," she mocked as she stuck her finger in the come, then licked it.

Robert didn't know what to do with himself.

For his final task, the Dom ordered Robert to get dressed, drive to a convenience store with the cum still on his face, take a photo with the clerk, and text it to him. It was 2 a.m. when Robert arrived at the nearest convenience store. He walked in, boldly approached the female clerk behind the counter, and asked if he could take a selfie with her. Surprisingly, she didn't mind or even ask him why. Robert quickly snapped the photo and sent it to the Dom.

Moments later his phone rang, and he heard the Dom and his wife laughing like hyenas on speakerphone. Apparently, neither of them expected he would do it and they were very impressed.

A few days later the Dom summoned Robert again.

"Meet me for lunch at the café down the block. Surprise me with a cool outfit," the Dom ordered.

Robert arrived at the café and found the Dom seated at a booth in the back. When he sat down, the Dom slid in beside him which seemed unusual.

"So, what outfit did you wear—show me. Go to the bathroom and text me pictures," he ordered.

Robert went to the single-occupancy restroom and jiggled the locked handle to ensure it was secure. He snapped photos of himself wearing a black velvet bra and matching panties over black fishnet stockings, texted them to the Dom, and then returned.

As they ordered their food, the Dom angled his cell phone so the waitress could see the photos Robert had sent him. Although she pretended not to notice, it was clear she did. Robert felt both humiliated and aroused but didn't say a word. The Dom didn't mention it either. They simply ate their burgers and drank a round of beer, avoiding any conversation about what had just happened.

A few weeks later, Robert returned to the Dom's house again. He was led down to the dungeon and ordered to stay there while the couple held a swinger's party upstairs. No one, except for the Dom and his wife, knew Robert was down there. Every now and then the Dom would sneak away from the guests and order Robert to service him with his mouth. Other times he came down and flogged Robert while he verbally humiliated him. That continued all night, and it wasn't until the last guest had left that Robert was finally allowed to leave.

They continued to hang out and over time Robert became much more comfortable with the Dom and his wife. He's now able to completely enjoy the evenings over at their place without hesitation. Before, Robert used to leave their house thinking *what the fuck did I just do?* but now he doesn't question himself at all. He also doesn't question his sexuality. He still considers himself straight and has zero attraction to men. But there's still just something about *his* Dom that's so mesmerizing to him. So mesmerizing that he continues to submit to him to this day.

Based on episode

511- Robert Is Hooking Up with a Male Dom Who Is Married

CONFESSION VIII: NEIL & RENEE

Neil and Renee are young, newbie swingers. So when did they decide to start swinging? Who did they start swinging with? And, how far do they go when swinging?

Already being open-minded people, it was easy for the couple to have candid discussions about their sexual fantasies. They used sex toys and frequently watched porn together. It never bothered Renee when Neil pointed out an attractive woman. On the contrary, it kind of turned her on. She questioned what specifically caught his attention. What did he like about her? Was it her ass or tits? The outfit she wore or the way she walked? In return, Renee felt empowered to tell Neil when she spotted a guy who aroused her interest. But that was as far as their risqué behavior went. They never had any intention of taking it further.

First Trip to a Swingers Resort

It was a regular evening just like any other when Renee and Neil were having some close neighborhood friends over for dinner. Perhaps it was the wine, or the fact that their friends couldn't keep things to themselves any longer, but secrets started to be revealed. Renee and Neil were floored to learn that their neighbors had been taking trips to a swinger resort for years. Neil and Renee, and the other vanilla couple dining with them, had lots of questions. With the help of the wine, the conversation flowed easily, and the back and forth continued until someone suggested that all three of the couples should take a trip to the resort together. A short debate ensued as to whether it would be wise to embark on such an adventure, but soon they threw caution to the wind and booked the tickets.

On arrival at the tropical destination, half-naked bodies aside, the resort itself was quite nice, and everyone was very friendly. It was slightly awkward at first seeing their female friends topless, but the community was so welcoming that they quickly settled into the vibe.

Neil and Renee decided to split off from their friends the first day and took an afternoon Boobs Cruise on a huge catamaran, with 150 other guests. As they left shore, the music was pumping, the drinks were flowing, and the clothes were starting to come off. The energy was palpable as everyone was dancing on the deck.

As crew members passed out drinks, the host shouted into the mic and asked who was ready to party. Everyone cheered as he promised it would be a trip to remember. The rowdy crowd, pumped with alcohol and energy, seemed ready to kick things up a notch, so the DJ asked if there were any squirters in the crowd. Two nude women raised their hands and were invited to lie down with their husbands kneeling beside them. A crowd gathered around to get a closer look at the brave volunteers.

The emcee explained he wanted to see how long it would take to make each contestant squirt before starting the countdown. Right on cue, the husbands vigorously fingered their wives, and within seconds, an explosion erupted resulting in a round of applause from the partygoers. Astonished by the presentation, the newbies couldn't fathom what other wild antics they would be lucky enough to witness. Renee, who thought squirting was a myth, was especially fascinated with the impressively messy display. The debaucherous games continued as the DJ requested the men to line up with the women standing before them. Numerous couples scrambled into position and awaited further instructions.

He momentarily paused the music to tell the women to give their men the best damn blow job possible. After he shouted "Go!" the party tunes kicked back on. Dropping to their knees, the ladies inhaled their partners' cocks. *Oh my God, what did we get ourselves into?* Neil and Renee wondered as they watched the porn-like scene of nearly forty simultaneous blow jobs play out in front of them. The entire cruise was nothing short of insane.

For the rest of their stay, they enjoyed the phenomenal people watching and tried to absorb the surreal environment. Obsessed by the world of sexual freedom, they made a commitment to learn more about it after they got back from the trip.

For the next several weeks after returning home, they tried to find resources online on how a couple should go about entering into the swinging scene. Sure, there were plenty of books on how to open up a marriage, but they wanted something less formal and in smaller bites. To their amazement, information was tough to come by. Eventually they gave up and went back to their satisfying yet vanilla sex life.

Venturing Further into the Lifestyle

Several weeks after the vacation, Renee confessed that she had grown bored with the vanilla, straight porn they had always been watching. Something inside her had been awakened and she wanted to see something different. They began watching threesome-themed porn, and Neil realized that Renee was overtly aroused during the girl-on-girl action. Broaching the subject, she confessed to having an experience with one of her female friends in college. The two coeds would share a hotel room when traveling, and on one particular night things unexpectedly heated up.

Renee said that upon returning to the room after a few drinks, the tipsy friend casually asked Renee to sit on her bed for a relaxing massage. Renee accepted the offer and before long, what started as an innocent back rub turned into the fondling of her breasts and both girls making out. Her friend then pushed Renee down on the bed, spread her legs and tasted her over and over again until she had one of the best orgasms of her life. She gladly returned the favor the next time they hooked up, and after that night, climbing into each other's bed became customary.

After telling Neil the story, Renee confessed that she wished she'd had more erotic encounters with women and wondered if perhaps the time had come. Neil suggested they could go to Vegas and get a woman for her, offering to just watch if she didn't want him to touch another woman. With the idea of opening their marriage on the table, they discussed the potential options: go to Vegas, or go back to the resort with their friends and commit to being more than voyeurs.

They returned to the adult resort with the other neighborhood couples as ready participants. They had a goal: find a woman for Renee to play with. Not wanting to confine themselves to any one thing, they were also open to other experiences if things transpired naturally. After making some new connections, they were invited to a hot tub with three other couples. The tub was fairly small, and the four ladies stripped down and hopped in first. The men gladly sat nearby and watched, each with a glass of whisky. Neil was in awe as he watched his wife caress and kiss the other women. When two of the couples abruptly left to fuck, Renee and the remaining woman decided to make their own plans.

They seductively told their husbands that they were taking it to the bedroom and both men followed. The heavy make-out session continued as the two women lay on the bed intertwined in each other's arms. Taking the lead, the other woman attended to every inch of Renee's body, making her feel at ease. Her touch was delicate and sensual. Renee liked the feel of her soft skin against hers and the smell of her floral perfume. The woman slowly kissed her neck and belly button as she inched her way lower down her body. Her mouth felt warm on Renee's pussy and her hair tickled Renee's inner thighs. After orgasming several times, they switched positions so Renee could have a taste as well. The woman's pussy was sweet and delicious as she came in her mouth. The only thing more amazing than going down on each other was the look on Neil's face as he watched from a corner of the room, enjoying the show.

After having their fill, the women invited the patient men to join. Renee unbuttoned Neil's pants on one side of the bed while the other couple played around right next to them. Respecting the boundaries of not touching each other's wives, the night ended with the couples having sex on the bed while right next to each other. It was a great first soft swap experience.

Neil and Renee were nothing but smiles as they said goodnight and departed for their own room. Wearing nothing but underwear and carrying armfuls of crumpled clothes, the giddy couple ended the night by fucking like crazy. Still high on adrenaline, they went at it again with each other the next morning. Hooking up in front of other people had been so thrilling and exciting for the first timers, it whetted their appetite for more.

As they triumphantly swapped stories with one of the other neighborhood couples, Neil and Renee learned they had also had a productive night. Similarly, the friends' evening started with them and another couple in a hot tub and ended with everyone exploring each other's bodies.

Hooking Up With the Neighbors

Upon arriving home after the vacation, the three couples were delighted with their progress and desperate for more. The couple who organized the trips were voyeurs, but the second couple was just as captivated by swinging as Neil and Renee. Unfortunately, a couple of months later the Covid-19 lockdown cramped their initial plans for future trips. Renee and Neil were disappointed that it was difficult to explore their newfound interests due to the pandemic, as were the second couple.

The two couples started taking daily afternoon walks together around the local lake, fantasizing about all the things they wanted to do when the world opened up again. Renee and the woman both wanted to continue their girl-on-girl journey which had barely started. When her friend suggested they should practice with each other, it seemed like the perfect way to receive feedback and build confidence in a safe space. After serious discussions about protecting the friendships, all four agreed it would be beneficial to play. Since the first couple was permanently stuck in the voyeur category due to the husband's jealousy issues, the four decided it would be best not to mention the experimental fun to avoid causing tension.

Later that night, Neil and Renee snuck out through their backyard, being careful not to be seen, and went to the second couple's house. At first, everyone was shy and unsure, and no one wanted to make the first move. Finally, the other husband suggested that the ladies take their clothes off. Granting the request, the women removed their tops and sat back on the couch. Pleased with their willingness to play along, Neil instructed them to start kissing. Again, the women happily obliged and began locking lips. The sexual excitement in the room began to build.

Watching the two ultra-attractive women get lost in each other was riveting for the two men. Still orchestrating the performance, they directed the women to go down on each other as they relished the live show before joining in on the action themselves. Neil went down on the other wife while Renee played with the other husband. Eventually everyone's bodies were intertwined in a fabulous pile.

Chatting afterward as they lie on the floor recovering, everyone felt surprisingly comfortable. The other couple wanted to know when they would be doing it again, and Neil and Renee asked what position they should try next.

Although most people considered the lockdown miserable, Neil and Renee found it unforgettably pleasurable. Each time they hooked up with the other couple, the group took turns sharing a fantasy that someone wanted to try. One wanted to fuck his wife from behind while she had her face buried in the other woman. One wanted to get fucked by her husband while the other wife licked her clit. Another wanted to receive a double blow job. Together they enthusiastically lived out each other's fantasies.

Each hook up was followed by a debrief the next day as they took their routine walk. The questions were always the same: What did you like? Did anything bother you? Is there anything you wish we hadn't done? Over the next few months, the foursome's sexual confidence blossomed with each new scenario. Even though they were having a wonderful time expanding their boundaries, hard swapping was still a bridge they weren't ready to cross.

Couple Swapping and More

After the pandemic subsided, Neil and Renee joined swinger websites to look for new play partners. They also attended house parties and hotel takeovers. During another group trip to the adult resort's new location in the Dominican Republic, they shared some more hot times with their favorite frisky neighbors after the voyeur couple had too much to drink one night.

With the stars aligned due to the voyeur couple's early departure, the four privately relaxed in the hot tub in Neil and Renee's room overlooking the beach. They took the party outside, and on the beach chairs, put on a show for people strolling by. Viewers could choose from watching Neil getting a blow job or Renee getting her pussy eaten with her legs spread wide open. The bystanders cheered and applauded.

Public sex was marvelous, and exhibitionism was quickly becoming a passion of theirs. Hearing random voices comment about the show they were putting on was an absolute highlight for Renee.

Then one evening, at the nightly party thrown by the adult resort, a very attractive Greek couple from the neighboring nude hotel approached Neil and Renee. The Greek man told Renee his wife thought she was really beautiful and was wondering what she would be like in bed. He then added that he thought Renee had the most breathtaking eyes. He confessed that he would love to make love to them.

Flattered, Neil and Renee accepted the proposition, and the four met the next evening. After a bit of dancing, they retired to Neil and Renee's room where they had drinks in the hot tub before moving to the bed, where the women got things started. The other woman was extremely vocal and sensual as Renee went down on her, continually moaning and begging for more with each orgasm.

Slowly, the other man kissed Renee's back as she made out with his wife. When he flipped her over, Neil took advantage of the moment and went down on the other wife while Renee was busy with the husband. Before they knew it, the mutual oral pleasuring gradually transitioned into full swapping, which they were surprisingly comfortable with. Everyone had a blast.

At the end of the night, Renee and Neil headed to the outdoor shower to reconnect. Knowing others could see their silhouettes through the glass turned them both on. Wanting to give the voyeurs something hot to look at, Renee told Neil to fuck her from behind as he pushed her up against the glass. Again, to their surprise, they heard cheers.

It was a night to remember, and they couldn't have asked for a cooler couple to pop their cherry with. Unfortunately, due to the distance, they never saw the Greek hotties again, but they certainly never forgot them.

Now, a few years later, Neil and Renee are a seasoned hard-swap couple who have perfected their script for playing. For them, they need to begin the evening with a little mingling and conversation before moving things to a more intimate setting. From there, Renee prefers the action to always start between the women before welcoming the men in. Having Neil watch her devour another woman turns both of them on and, ideally, the evening will end with the two couples hard swapping. But regardless of how the night goes, reconnecting with each other at the end of the date is the most important and rewarding part.

Thinking back to how lost they felt when they first entered into the lifestyle, they decided to build a website to help other newbies, as well as seasoned folks looking for additional information. They soon launched their website, Tempted Pineapples. On it you can find party ideas, swinger dating websites, sex toy reviews, lists of adult resorts, and plenty more.

Above all, their journey into the wild world of swinging has been a wonderful experience. Aside from the wild sex, they love the judgment-free attitude and complementary nature of swingers. They truly feel they have found their people.

Based on episodes

628 - Neil and His Wife Started Swinging with Their Neighbors, and They Have All Been Swinging Ever Since

637 - Renee and Her Husband Started Swinging with Their Neighbors, and They've Been Swinging Ever Since

Their website can be found here: https://www.temptedpineapples.com

CONFESSION IX: KYLE

As a recent divorcé, Kyle was determined to take full advantage of his newly acquired freedom and fulfill some of his wildest, unresolved fantasies. From being monogamous and married to entering into the lifestyle as a single, older guy, Kyle experienced swinging, being a cuck, gang bangs, and more.

The First Couple

Kyle spent most of his adult life monogamously married and always wondered how the other side lived. When he got divorced in his early sixties, he knew he didn't want to jump into a monogamous relationship. Instead, he decided to sow his wild oats and explore the lifestyle. His first hook up was with a couple he met on Craigslist who were looking to have threesomes. When he arrived at their house a six-foot-five man answered the door and Kyle immediately thought, *what the fuck did I get myself into?*

Soon after he walked in, the man's wife, a very sexy blonde wearing a skimpy sundress, appeared and put Kyle at ease. After what seemed like only ten minutes of being at the house, to his surprise, the horny housewife got on the pool table, and with her dress scrunched up around her waist, invited Kyle in for a taste. Kyle got down on his knees in front of her and stared at his first new pussy in thirty years. As Kyle began to go to work on her, she wrapped her long legs around his head and squeezed her thighs each time his tongue licked her clit.

To Kyle's amazement, the husband just sat there and watched, while he stroked his cock; it was obvious he was enjoying the scene. He instructed his wife to be a good hostess and give their guest some extra attention. The wife hopped off the pool table, knelt in front of Kyle, and slowly unbuckled his pants. Kyle was on fire as she took his cock out and put it in her mouth. As she skillfully went to work on him, the husband bragged about his wife's exceptional oral skills and kept asking Kyle if she was doing a good job.

Kyle was experiencing so much ecstasy he was barely able to mutter a reply. Her mouth, tongue, and hand worked in perfect harmony as she repeatedly brought him to the brink of orgasm before abruptly stopping. *If the foreplay is this phenomenal, imagine how good the sex will be,* Kyle thought. When the trio finally moved to a bedroom that was specifically reserved for hosting playdates, Kyle noticed cameras had been set up.

Being filmed for the couple didn't bother Kyle at all—in fact, it was a huge turn-on for him. He was an exhibitionist at heart. As they got onto the bed, the husband finally joined in on the action and for the next hour and a half, the three of them went at it. At one point, while the wife was riding Kyle, her husband slid into her ass. Kyle had officially participated in his first double penetration; he couldn't believe he was acting out something he had only ever seen in porn—on his first night of swinging no less. After hooking up with them a handful of times, Kyle was hooked on MFM (male-female-male) threesomes and decided to go find as many couples as he could to have some more.

The Next Couple

Kyle's next hookup was with a couple in their late fifties. The husband was a wealthy stockbroker, and the wife was a secretary, but when it came to sex, they enjoyed switching things up. Exchanging power roles, the wife morphed into the dominant partner who got everything she wanted, and the husband was only there to observe. They initially met at a rooftop bar in Fort Lauderdale where the three of them sat down in a booth with Kyle, the wife on one side, and the husband on the other.

Immediately, the wife's hands were all over Kyle and soon they were making out. The exhibitionist in Kyle got super aroused when she took his hand and put it up her loose skirt so he could slide his fingers into her. The husband smiled as he sat across from them watching the action. Soon she suggested to Kyle that they get out of there and told her husband to take them for a drive. Kyle agreed without hesitation.

Kyle and the wife fell into the back seat of the car, and the husband got into the driver's seat. As they began to slowly cruise around town, Kyle and the man's wife were all over each other, and soon she had her shirt off and his pants wide open. With her long fingers wrapped around his rock-hard cock and her bare breasts firmly pressed against him, she whispered in his ear: "I can't wait to have all of you in my mouth."

Kyle glanced over and saw the husband watching in the rear-view mirror as she lowered her head and took all of Kyle deep into her throat. He could barely contain himself as she deep throated him in the back seat of the car. Finally, he couldn't take it any longer. And just when he was about to explode, the wife took him out of her mouth and aggressively started jacking him off, directing the spray all over her naked breasts. Kyle sat back and marveled at how hot her tits looked with his cum all over them. To his amazement, she then leaned toward the front seat and told her husband to lick her tits clean.

Not only was the sex hot as fuck with those two, Kyle also found that he really liked them. As the three started to become closer friends, Kyle realized the couple was extremely well connected in the Florida swinging scene. They knew about all the different swinger events and clubs in the area, and it turned out they also hosted their own swinger parties. The first one they invited Kyle to was a Big Black Cock party which they hosted several times a year in a rented mansion.

When he arrived at the two-day event and entered into the main room of the couples' mansion, he saw a naked crowd of about thirty Black men and around ten white couples. As Kyle walked around, he saw various sex acts going down throughout the mansion. At the top of the staircase, on the landing, he saw a woman wearing nothing but a pair of stiletto heels being pounded by two well built, well-hung Black men. Her husband was right next to them stroking himself as he watched the scene unfold.

In another spot he saw two hot white women going at it with two Black men on a huge mattress in the middle of the floor. He eventually stumbled into a room and watched a single woman being aggressively fucked by three Black men with huge cocks. While one was fucking her, another was holding her head and fucking her mouth while the third was rubbing his BBC on her breasts. Of course, her husband stood on the sidelines and watched.

Kyle was initially overwhelmed. But soon, his horniness took over and he approached a sexy topless woman who was standing on her own. After he asked her if she wanted to play, the woman politely responded that she had already been with eight different guys that evening and was taking a well-deserved break. *Oh my God, it's only nine o'clock,* he thought. As they continued to chat, a man wearing a fanny pack filled with lube, wipes, and condoms joined the conversation. It was her husband. Apparently, his job was to provide condoms and lube to the men as they fucked her. Later that evening, Kyle watched the pair in action. As she got rocked by four more huge Black men, it became clear she had a preference for them.

The Librarian

Though Kyle ended up only being a voyeur at that first BBC party, he still had an amazing time. For the next few events, Kyle brought dates with him, instead of going solo, which completely changed the dynamic. One of his first dates was with a forty-two-year-old woman he met on a vanilla dating site who looked like a librarian. Although Kyle could tell she was open-minded sexually, he had no idea how much she would eagerly embrace the swinger lifestyle. But within minutes of arriving at her first party, his date turned to Kyle and whispered, "Let's go fuck," and then led him to an empty bedroom.

As the two of them were going at it, they were interrupted by a naked man who politely asked if he could join them. Kyle looked at his date who nodded, then watched as she reached out, grabbed the man's cock and started blowing him. Kyle was in ecstasy as he continued to fuck her. This was the first time he had ever shared a woman that *he* was dating, and it was mind blowing.

Suddenly, a younger guy in his early twenties joined in and she took turns blowing the two of them. Then another man showed up and Kyle stepped aside. He watched in awe as she played with the three Black men over the course of an hour. Occasionally, he jumped in, but mostly he just enjoyed watching her repeatedly orgasm from the multitude of men. It was then that he realized he just might be a cuck.

On their way home, Kyle asked her what she had thought of the night's events. Without pausing, she devilishly responded: "When's the next party?"

Kyle continued to casually date the hypersexual hottie and couldn't believe how insatiable she was. On the way home from the supermarket, she would slide her pants off and masturbate in the car to see how many orgasms she could have before arriving back home. *Geez, it's only four miles! It's not even worth it, can't you just wait?* Kyle always wondered.

The sexy surprises continued when Kyle took her to her first swinger's club. Within thirty minutes of being inside, his date was spread-eagle on a barstool getting eaten out by a woman. A small crowd had gathered around to watch the two beautiful lingerie-clad ladies. The hot scene got even more intense when he discovered she was a squirter, drenching the woman's face and matting her hair. He immediately grabbed her, bent her over the bar stool, and fucked her in front of everyone.

The hot and steamy times with the sexy librarian-looking woman continued for the next few months but eventually they parted ways.

Newly Naughty Doreen

After splitting up with the "librarian," Kyle fell into a committed relationship with a woman named Doreen and continued to explore his new role as the cuck. Kyle made it a point to be open and honest with her about his sexual history and interests before meeting her in person. He explained that he was not only into swinging, but he also had recently been turned on to the cuckold dynamic.

Thankfully, his kinky confession did not scare her away. Instead, she was slightly intrigued. For the next six months, they had multiple conversations, and she spent time researching things like MFM (male-female-male) threesomes and cuckolding. Finally ready to test her naughty side, the couple created a profile on an adult dating site and Doreen quickly selected a guy she was attracted to.

After exchanging numbers, the three chatted in a group text which soon escalated to sexting. Kyle got aroused reading the flirtatious messages between Doreen and the online hottie. One night, Kyle came home, and Doreen had exciting news: "He wants to meet us tonight!"

Kyle was down and so was Doreen. At five o'clock, they met at a local bar. When the online hot guy walked in, they were both happy; he was even hotter in person. With Doreen sitting between them, both men's hands wandered under her dress and up her legs. Kyle continued to rub her thigh as the man slid his fingers inside Doreen. Seeing her smile, Kyle decided to go to the bar to give them privacy. Watching from a distance, he noticed that the bartenders could also see what was happening and were thrilled.

When he returned to the table, he saw that Doreen was rubbing the man's cock through his pants. She seductively whispered to Kyle that he was rock hard and suggested that it was time to get a room. Walking into the hotel lobby with both men's arms wrapped around her, it was obvious to the staff what was going to happen. Knowing other people could tell his date was about to get fucked by two guys drove Kyle wild. The horny trio headed to the room and once inside, to Kyle's surprise, Doreen took over. She pointed to Kyle and instructed him to sit on the bed.

Next, she looked at the other guy and ordered him to sit in a chair. Once she had arranged everyone in their proper places, Doreen lowered to her knees, removed the other man's pants, and began slowly sucking on him as Kyle watched. Kyle was getting extremely aroused and started undressing.

"No, no, no! You just get to watch!" Doreen shouted, putting Kyle in place.

Doreen proceeded to passionately blow the guy while refusing to allow Kyle to participate or even touch himself. Kyle couldn't believe how hot it was to be at her mercy. He then watched as the other man led his girlfriend to the bed and devoured her. It was magnificent.

Doreen then told the man to lay down on the bed. As she climbed on top of him, she grabbed his cock, rubbed it against her clit, and let it glide inside her. It was so visually satisfying that Kyle nearly exploded in his pants. At that moment it became apparent that Doreen loved cuckolding as much as Kyle loved being cuckolded.

With Doreen eager to fuck more guys and Kyle eager to push his cuck fantasy even further, Kyle arranged a playdate with an acquaintance who he knew was precisely Doreen's type. He chose a hotel located in a remote section of South Miami as the perfect spot. When the day arrived, and he introduced the acquaintance to Doreen, it was the first time she had ever seen or spoken to him. For Kyle, this just added another spicy element to the encounter.

From the mirrored ceilings and walls to the see-through shower, the room appeared to have been designed for sex, which helped set the mood. As the three sat and chatted, the bull asked Doreen if he could kiss her. With permission granted, he leaned in and made out with Doreen as Kyle watched. Thoroughly turned on, Kyle gently reached down and guided her legs open. Understanding the signal, the bull automatically lowered to his knees and started gingerly licking her before diving deeper in with his tongue.

"Oh my God, no one has ever eaten my pussy like this before!" she exclaimed as her body convulsed.

As she squirmed and screamed with delight, Kyle sat back and filmed the glorious action.

"Holy shit, I love the way he's devouring me," she repeatedly shouted in between gasping breaths.

"I hope you are taking notes because you could learn a thing or two!"

Her feisty attitude made his cock throb. The lively dirty talk continued as he turned to fuck her doggy-style. All the while she couldn't stop raving about how deep he was and how amazing it felt.

Doreen finally allowed Kyle to undress and join in. They each took a turn licking her pussy and fucking her, and they ended the evening by double penetrating her. The threesome was so much fun that they met up with the bull five more times.

Doreen constantly kept Kyle on his toes. One morning he awoke to discover Doreen's vibrator and dildo on the kitchen counter. Beside the come-covered toys, was a note that read: *I called our bull last night and he got me off over the phone. Now it's your job to lick these clean.*

While at work one day, he received a text from Doreen telling him someone was coming over for dinner. When he opened the front door, Kyle was greeted by Doreen sitting on the dining room table as their bull was going down on her. The glow of the dimly lit chandelier made her look ethereal. As he fucked her for several hours, Kyle's attempts to join in were repeatedly rejected. As Doreen was busy, Kyle just sat there and stroked himself until she was done. It wasn't until the other guy orgasmed that Kyle was allowed to enjoy her.

Kyle and Doreen continued to date for the next couple of months but unfortunately their steamy relationship eventually ended, and Kyle began looking for his next dating adventure.

Stacey, the Horny School Teacher

Next, Kyle met Stacey, a second-grade school teacher in her mid-thirties, whom he also met on a mainstream dating site. He quickly found out she loved to get fucked a lot, but she had never participated in a gang bang and wanted to. Kyle suggested she join him at a private swinger party where a gang bang could easily be arranged. Stacey was on board with the plan.

The swinger event was hosted by his friends, the same couple who had hosted the BBC parties. This event was a hotwife party, designed to ensure that the women got whatever and whoever they wanted. The party consisted of around fifty Black men and about fifteen hotwives. Unlike their previous parties, this one was thrown in a warehouse that was decked out with beds and classy decorations everywhere. The entire place pumped with energy as orgies and gang bangs took place throughout the room.

Stacey sat on one of the beds, and within minutes she had five Black men all over her. The men helped her out of her clothes and laid her down. With meticulous care they went to work on every part of her body. Slowly the five men enveloped her until Kyle could only hear her moans. After quite a bit of time without even catching so much as a glimpse of her, Kyle wanted to make sure she was okay. He called out: "Stacey! Are you all right?"

Suddenly from the mass of Black men, a little white arm popped out and gave him a thumbs up, then quickly disappeared. Kyle laughed and thought to himself, *I can't believe this is my life.* Kyle continues to see Stacey and they've been back to that event many times together.

Even though Kyle has already experienced so much in the lifestyle he has no plans to stop any time soon. Having experimented with threesomes, cuckolding, gang bangs, and more he sometimes wonders if he'll ever be able to be in a traditional relationship again.

Though he's not really sure what the answer is, he's also not worried about it. In his sixties he's finally living his best life and looks forward to even more crazy experiences.

Based on episode

812 - Kyle Is a Swinger into Cuckolding, Gang Bangs, Hotwifing, and More

CONFESSION X: CASEY

As a unicorn in the lifestyle, Casey had access to an abundance of men. When she journeyed into the world of gang bangs at a friend's suggestion, the ability to maximize the number of guys she could juggle at once became a dream come true.

Soon after venturing into the lifestyle, Casey quickly racked up numerous MF (Male-Female) and MFM (male-female-male) encounters. Noticing how insatiable she was becoming, one of her regular playmates offered to host a gang bang to feed Casey's desire. Her friend was a seasoned swinger with a vast list of available guys. Although she initially passed, Casey eventually accepted, since she was getting bored with only having two guys at a time. The truth was she had way more energy and stamina than her partners. A lot of the time the guys were exhausted before she even broke a sweat. She decided it was finally the right time to expand her repertoire, and told her friend she was ready to have a gang bang.

Challenged at Her First Gang Bang

Her friend said he'd take care of everything and all she needed to do was be ready at 7 p.m. that Saturday. He'd pick her up and take her to a secret location, she would have her fun with a few guys, and then they would leave. He made it sound so simple and easy with nothing to worry about. Knowing he had had previous experience being a gang bang coordinator for other female playmates, she trusted him and didn't ask for specific details. Embracing the spontaneity, she put her faith in him.

The secret arrangement was unusual for Casey. She literally had no idea what town or place they were meeting in. It was unusual for her, and she was a little nervous. Normally, she maintained control of the details and always met up with the suitors in a public place before fucking. It was the first time she just showed up to a mysterious location with guys ready to fuck her, already there, with no prior interaction.

As they pulled up to the secret location, the pressure was on. She paused and took a few deep breaths, before getting out of the car. The front door was unlocked, and they just walked right in which felt odd to her. Her friend, who was now in his role as the coordinator, told her to change into her lingerie. He then escorted her to a back bedroom where four Black men were waiting for her. There was no banter or name exchange, and the businesslike vibe produced a mix of emotions for her. As she stood in the room surrounded by a bunch of unfamiliar faces, she tried to remain calm.

One of the guys asked for her safe word, and arrogantly explained that she was going to need it. Her emotions exploded. *How dare this guy challenge me; who the fuck does he think he is?* she thought. The only thing Casey hated more than being self-conscious was being doubted. It fueled a fire deep inside her.

"I'll give you a word, but I guarantee you, I won't be using it."

With Casey welcoming the challenge, they immediately got down to business. There was no background music or lighthearted side conversations which helped make the vibe focused and ultraserious. The first guy bent her over the edge of the bed and started in on her aggressively. When he tired of the high energy fucking, another would instantly take his place and continue the pounding, with the first guy resting on the side till it was his turn again.

Around and around, they went on her, with the intensity never letting up. To their amazement Casey continued to take it all. Fueled by her competitive nature, any lack of confidence she was hiding began to fall away and she got stronger with each new guy.

After several rounds of her pussy getting beaten with the monster cocks, and no cry of her safe word, they teamed up. First, they added hard face fucking while she was getting slammed from behind. When she took that in stride, they forced a double vaginal on her. Still, she took it. Then all four went to work on her with a double vaginal and a double face fucking simultaneously, forcing her body to contort to take the punishment. Casey felt like a prize fighter in the ring, taking hit after hit but refusing to get knocked down.

For three hours Casey was pounded by four guys trying to destroy her, and the impact on her body was intense. However, it was more than just a physical fight: it was a mental battle. It was her will against theirs, an endurance test to see who would tap out first. Determined to be victorious, Casey refused to surrender. Finally, when all the men were exhausted and depleted, she was the last one standing.

"Holy shit, who is this girl?" one of the guys muttered.

Their admiration and shock had Casey feeling a level of empowerment far superior to anything she had ever felt before. She decided, from that moment on, there would be no limit to how many cocks she could outlast.

With the night a success, her interest in gang bangs was sparked. To savor the memory, she abstained from sex for the next few days. She needed time to let the gravity of her achievement settle in. She wanted to fully appreciate it. Ironically, her pussy was not even sore, but her abs were on fire from bracing herself all night. Starring in the gang bang had been the equivalent of a full-body workout.

Arranging Her Own Gang Bangs

Casey knew some people thought of gang bangs as trashy and demeaning, but that's not how she viewed it. Not only was it an empowering experience for her, she saw them as the perfect opportunity to have all her desires filled in one night. Double vaginal penetration; spit roasting; double blow jobs: she welcomed it all. Where else but at a gang bang could she have two cocks in her pussy and two more in her mouth at the same time?

She wanted her friend to set another one up for her, but he wasn't immediately able to do so. As an independent woman, she hated relying on other people and decided to take matters into her own hands. *I'm a smart girl, I can figure this out,* she figured.

Curating her own gang bangs allowed Casey to handpick her men: good looking guys with big dicks. It was simple to post ads for participants and get hundreds of responses, but getting the exact right mix of guys was time consuming and she never really knew if it would work well till they were all together. New guys were a double-edged sword. They posed the risk of flaking or having stage fright, but the unknown nature added some mystery, and sometimes newbies turned out to be the superstars. Good performers from previous gang bangs were dependable but had already showcased their skills so they were less exciting. For that reason, Casey preferred a blend of wildcard newbies and seasoned regulars.

Of course, just because a guy was a hot piece of eye candy did not mean he would turn out to be a valuable gang bang guy. An open-minded attitude, excellent stamina, the ability to play well with others, and the willingness to cross swords were the qualities she looked for in a guy. Some guys were curious about the group atmosphere but would panic when another guy's cock got too close to theirs. She especially appreciated guys who went above and beyond in the teamwork category. Guys who manually held two cocks together for her hungry mouth or took the initiative to help reinsert another cock during a double vaginal mishap held a special place in her heart.

Soon she was curating gang bangs for herself every week, with five to seven guys, lasting three to four hours. Sometimes she instructed everyone to show up at the same time and other times she staggered their arrivals. The ultimate goal was to never be without a hard cock ready to fill her. Nothing was worse than a gang bang where all the guys needed to recover at the same time, which shut down the vibe and left her pussy empty. Either way, there were never any guarantees about how the night would develop. Would all the guys show up? Would they all be able to perform? How long would they last? The list of questions was long, but the unknown element of gang bangs became part of the allure for her.

Although she loved the high-adrenaline stakes of multiple guys, Casey understood the need for safety. Logistically, she couldn't keep an eye on everything with a bunch of cocks in her face, so for each gang bang, she always had a loyal friend to act as security. Duties ranged from supplying condoms, answering the door for latecomers, and most importantly making sure no one got out of hand. Her nightly "bodyguard" was always a voyeuristic partner who had a kink for used pussy, and gladly waited until the end of the night to have his turn with her.

Eventually, word spread of Casey's gang bangs, and she had a waiting list of guys dying to get an invite. While hotel gatherings were in a controlled environment, public gang bangs at swinger clubs offered a completely different experience. She would attend clubs on single-guy nights, and post her whereabouts online; not knowing how many guys would show up was part of the fun. On a slow night, she might only fuck one guy, but on a busier night, it could be a dozen or more. Getting pummeled by a line of guys was more about them getting off than Casey being pampered.

Since the clientele was random at the clubs, she implemented stricter rules like no kissing or oral, and loosened her requirements for physical attraction since it was more about the guys performing a function for her. During visits when she was on the hunt and didn't like the available options from an aesthetic point of view, blindfolds became an invaluable tool. Removing her sight allowed her to imagine the cock inside her belonged to whatever dream hunk she wanted. She also found that losing one sense heightened the others, which created an altered sensation and led to great orgasms.

Gang Bangs and Her Personal Life

Just as the guys could not be properly judged by appearance, neither could Casey. Clothed, she behaved shy and quiet, but as soon as she got naked, she morphed into a savage animal ready to attack. The only downside to Casey's undeniable passion for cock was it created a frustrating problem for her love life. Unfortunately, her gang bang hobby deterred several potential boyfriends from pursuing a serious relationship with her. A few even had the audacity to say she needed to be monogamous to settle down with them, even though they met in the lifestyle. She frequently wondered: *Is there something wrong with me? Will anyone ever accept me for who I truly am?*

Luckily, when Casey met her husband, she no longer had to question if she had to give up who she was and what she desired. Not only did he support her insatiable appetite, he constantly pushed her to be a bigger slut. Since they were initially introduced during a threesome, sharing her with other men was natural to him and they slowly transitioned into a stag/vixen relationship. When planning a date with somebody new, he would often comment: "Why only one guy? Why not get three? Hell, why not find five?"

Unexpectedly, her love of gang bangs wound up benefiting their relationship. When they were alone, her husband constantly worried that he was hurting her during the rough sex she liked to have. But for some reason, when other men were added to the scene, her husband automatically flipped a switch and became an alpha Dom with no remorse. He embraced the mob mentality and fed off the other men's energy, commanding them to do his bidding.

"Use this little 'whore,'" he would say and then stand back and proudly watch her get pummeled.

But beyond his help with the operational aspect of her gang bangs, he provided a safe environment where she felt comfortable letting her guard down and pushing her boundaries. They started incorporating new elements like hardcore face-fucking blow jobs, being leashed and collared, and excessive dirty talk with vulgar name calling. As her stag, he earned the privilege to choose her dates according to what he wanted. If there was a fetish or sex act he had been fantasizing about, she happily integrated it during playtime to appease him. Although she adopted certain submissive behaviors, Casey always maintained her dominant attitude. Even when collared, she taunted and mocked the guys: "Is that all you got?"

Although anonymous sex was her kink, her sociable husband preferred a more connected experience with the men. As a compromise, they alternated between meeting the guys in the hotel room and meeting them downstairs for a drink first. Being an experienced single male in the lifestyle himself, her husband was sympathetic to the men and always rooted for them to succeed with his wife. She found it endearing when he acted as their coach, giving them pep talks when they had erection issues and offering tips on how to satisfy her. Given that guys often got a bad rap for being thirsty or disgusting, they always appreciated having him as an ally. After all, without single guys, Casey wouldn't be able to do what she loved so much, and nothing made her husband smile more than when Casey was fully satisfied.

Her Cum Fetish

In addition to her gang bang addiction, Casey also had a huge cum fetish. Unfortunately, her husband was not as keen on cum play as she was, but gang bangs provided the solution. It was simple math to her—the more guys there were, the more cum she could receive. After a killer gang bang, she expected to be a sticky mess. A glorious cum shot was the epitome of a job well done for the cum queen. Without it, even an award-winning performance would be considered anticlimactic. For her, the epic sticky grand finale was one of the most important parts of an experience.

Although guys were required to wear condoms at her gang bangs, she always insisted they come on her body so she could enjoy the sensation of it against her bare skin. Fascinated by the texture, she liked to rub it all over her body and admired guys who didn't mind getting dirty with her. If one guy shot a load on her and then another guy fucked her with his hand firmly planted in it, she was elated. While a man touching someone else's cum was hot, nothing drove her crazier than a guy who liked to taste it. Though it occasionally happened, that level of dedication was much harder to come by.

After some fifty or sixty gang bangs the girl who cherished the moments of her first gang bang in solitude gradually disappeared. Now, after getting wrecked for hours with no breaks, Casey was instantly ready for more. You might assume a girl would be exhausted by then, but the endless orgasms only made her hornier. Each time all of the cocks were sufficiently drained and the guests left, Casey turned to her husband with a devilish look in her eye.

"It's your turn now."

Based on episodes

527 - Casey Is a Vixen into Swinging, DV, Gang Bangs, and More
548 - Casey Has Been in Over 50 Gang Bangs
Her OnlyFans: https://onlyfans.com/hotwifelife869

CONFESSION XI: MARA

Mara married her high school sweetheart and as a result assumed that her long-time, secret fantasy of being with a woman would remain unfulfilled. She never could have possibly dreamed that after nearly twenty years of a vanilla marriage, her wish would be granted, and a generous hall pass would turn into a polyamorous love triangle.

Mara's bi-curiosity was obvious to her from a young age. The first crush she could remember was one she had on a girl. She had made out with a few girls when she was young, and it always left her wanting more. Eventually, Mara ended up on a more traditional path and got married to a man at a fairly young age. But she never let go of her attraction to women. Mara constantly thought about being with women when she masturbated and even occasionally did it while fucking her husband.

Throughout the years, she was tempted to confide in him several times, but her fear of judgment and rejection always stopped her. After keeping her desire a secret for so long, the thirty-seven-year-old finally came to a realization: life was short and she didn't want to die without having the experience of being with a woman—it was time to let him know.

At first, she started by subtly dropping hints, jokingly telling him that if he let her have a girlfriend, she wouldn't be so needy. But the casual comments didn't grab his attention. So, one morning she finally blurted it out.

"I really want to fuck a girl."

Unfortunately, it didn't go as she'd hoped. Much to her surprise, the thought of his wife with another woman did not interest her husband. Although he did not approve of the abrupt announcement, it did at least open the door to an honest conversation. After some discussion, he told her maybe he would be open to it at some point, but not at that moment.

The Free Pass

For the next several months, Mara continued to bring up the topic but made no progress. When a coworker told Mara about a cool app where users could find people who were into all kinds of nontraditional arrangements, she wanted to check it out. She asked her husband if he would mind if she created an account just to look and after a lot of discussion, he agreed. His conditions were that she could only use it to look and they would need to talk more if she ever wanted to take things further.

Fascinated by the hook-up app, she spent hours scrolling through female profiles. When Mara found a woman's profile that piqued her interest, she asked her husband for permission to meet up with her. Since the woman she liked was also married, he was open to it and surprisingly gave her a hall pass. He told her he was okay with her having a "friend with benefits," but *one* was enough. He didn't want her sleeping with a bunch of different women. He was hoping she'd pursue her fantasy just one time, and be done with it.

Mara agreed, immediately reached out to the woman, and they started chatting. Mara's initial attraction was purely physical, but the more they talked, she discovered that she also liked the woman as a person. Their conversations were fun and easy, and soon the two nonmonogamous newbies felt like they had been friends for a long time. It turned out they also had a lot in common. They were both around the same age, had been with their partners since high school, and decided to open their relationships up at around the same time. The only difference was that the other woman identified as a lesbian and was married to a woman.

The night before they arranged to meet in person for the first time, it was obvious Mara's husband was having a tough time with it all. Seeing him so emotional and scared, made her realize that having a fling was not worth risking her marriage. She offered to cancel the date and stop talking to her new friend, but her husband refused. He told her he loved her and didn't want to be the one to stop her from doing something she wanted, possibly even needed, to do.

The next day, she was extremely nervous waiting at the coffee shop for her date. When her new friend walked in, she was thrilled to see that she was even better looking in person. Both women were slightly awkward at first as they chatted over coffee, but the conversation eventually found its rhythm. As they continued to talk and flirt with each other Mara started wondering what it would be like to kiss her.

When they walked out to the parking lot to say goodbye, Mara couldn't resist and suggested a make out session. The woman eagerly nodded and stepped closer to her. Mara was both excited and nervous as she placed her hands on the woman's waist and slowly pulled her in. When their lips finally touched, the moment felt explosive. Their hips fit together so perfectly that she completely sunk into the sensation of the woman's body pressed against hers. It was so sensual, so natural, so *different* from what she was used to. Their physical chemistry was undeniable, and the thrill was addictive. They knew they were going to have to see each other again soon.

Their connection was easy. They met for drinks often and went on shopping trips together, sometimes sneaking quick make out sessions in changing rooms. Eventually, the sexual tension built up and they realized it had to be released. So, for Mara's birthday, the woman rented a house for a sexy celebration.

"I'm going to lose my lesbian virginity tonight," Mara told her husband as she was getting ready for the big night. Although Mara's husband did not want to know every little detail about her escapades, he appreciated being kept in the loop and was genuinely excited for her.

To prepare for the big event, Mara got her first Brazilian wax so she would be silky smooth. As she drove to the rental, she was buzzing with anticipation. The butterflies in her stomach were all part of the fun for her. When she got there and they were finally alone, their conversation had a nervous quality to it. Mara noticed her new friend was just as anxious as she was, which ironically calmed her down and made her feel more comfortable.

They quickly decided to move into the bedroom. Mara sat on the edge of the bed as her friend began to touch her. It was intoxicating to smell her perfume and to feel her hands slowly caress her body. Mara had never been with a woman beyond kissing and closed her eyes as she let the woman's hands explore. Soon she was pulling Mara's blouse up over her head and then Mara returned the favor. As the two sat there in their bras, Mara reached out to hold the woman's breasts in both her hands. Then she gently ran her finger over the top, tracing her curves before reaching both hands behind and releasing her bra. Her bare breasts were so beautiful and soft that Mara felt enchanted by the woman's body. She lowered her head to take one breast in her mouth and after a quick kiss of her nipples, her lover pushed her back onto the bed and got on top of her. She pressed Mara down and kissed her with fiery passion. Slowly the woman worked her way lower, kissing her body the entire way. She pulled Mara's skirt off, moved her panties out of the way, and tasted her properly.

Having never felt anything like it before, Mara gasped at the sensation. It was a woman licking her. It was a woman with her fingers inside her. It was a woman that was about to make her come. She grabbed a pillow, mashed it down on her face, and screamed into it as her body exploded. She experienced one of the most powerful orgasms she had ever had, even more thrilling than she had ever expected.

For two hours the pair played with each other and orgasmed over, and over, and over again. At times it was soft and gentle, and other times it was rough; rougher than her husband had ever been with her, and she liked it. When they'd both had enough, they got dressed and headed home for the night since neither was allowed to sleep over. As Mara drove away from the property, the fact that they had just used it for their lesbian lovefest only added to the hotness of the evening for her.

From that night on, they fell into a routine. They met for coffee during the week and then met on the weekend to play. The pair were having incredible sex, but Mara realized the casual hookup was becoming more serious and emotions were developing between them. To further complicate things, the woman admitted that her marriage was starting to suffer. That left Mara feeling guilty and she wondered if they should end things. She felt bad that the women's relationship was being negatively affected because she was having the exact opposite experience in her marriage.

Her Bi-Exploration

As a result of exploring her lesbian side, Mara and her husband's sex life only got better. After seeing her lover, she always returned home super turned on. The minute she'd walk in she'd throw her husband down and ride him until he came. She found herself more attracted to him. There was something about him allowing her to indulge in her fantasy that made him even sexier and more desirable to her.

In an effort to not take their marriage for granted, they decided to make every Thursday night date night. Thursday night dates soon turned into Thursday night fuckfests, which then fueled her weekend encounters with her lesbian lover. And, that in turn fueled her desire for her husband. It was an added benefit that neither Mara nor her husband could have expected.

To Mara, the craziest part of her bi-exploration, however, was discovering how much she loved going down on a woman. She considered herself a pillow princess within her marriage and always hated giving a blow job. Unexpectedly, eating pussy quickly became a favorite hobby of hers. It certainly didn't hurt that her girlfriend was blessed with an adorable pussy that Mara found irresistible. Plus, the soft sounds her lover made when orgasming were music to her ears. Seeing her skin flush and feeling her hips writhe while Mara ate her pussy was better than any experience she'd ever had in bed.

Mara was so happy enjoying the both of them that she hoped to arrange a threesome with her husband and her lover, but neither was overly keen on the idea. Her lover preferred to keep Mara for herself at the moment and the husband wasn't the type to sleep with someone he was not in a committed relationship with. So for the time being, Mara enjoyed the both of them separately, and assumed things would just stay that way.

One thing that Mara was curious about and couldn't wait to try was strap-on play. They had talked about it several times, and to Mara, it sounded really hot. Getting to fuck a woman with a cock was something Mara wanted to experience. Unfortunately, on the night it was set to go down, her girlfriend showed up crying.

"We can't see each other for a whole month," she sobbed.

The relationship with her wife had finally reached the breaking point and the wife insisted that they take a break. Mara felt blind-sided. As she sat there devastated, unsure of what to do next, she realized that her feelings for her girlfriend were far stronger than she had known.

That night, Mara cried herself to sleep. As the tears continued the next morning, her husband, in true fashion, was there to support her. As the month passed, the radio silence was unbearable. She felt a huge void without the daily conversations she had grown accustomed to with her close friend and lover. Unable to control herself, Mara broke the rules and sent a message but got no response. Then a few days later, the phone rang and it was her. She told Mara that her wife was threatening to extend their separation.

Mara was wrecked: the not knowing when they would be reunited was brutal. She desperately wanted something concrete to hold on to. A date she could look forward to was all she felt she needed. Surprisingly, only three days later, Mara received a text from her lover. It read: *My wife and I are getting a divorce.*

The Threesome

Although Mara felt guilty about her girlfriend's divorce, she was excited that they were going to be able to see each other again.

Mara was thrilled to be reunited with her lover. She even fulfilled her bucket list goal of using a strap-on, which was mind-blowingly fun. Mara was in heaven as they took turns fucking each other with the dildo. Mara found she preferred wearing it versus receiving it. She loved being the more dominant partner, a role that she had never held before.

Their relationship continued to progress, and Mara was ecstatic when her lover invited her on a trip to California. When her husband saw how excited she was, although it was against the rules, he couldn't say no. During the week-long girls-only trip, Mara enjoyed being an official couple with her girlfriend for the first time. Far from home, with no possibility of bumping into someone she knew, Mara relaxed and fully immersed herself in every moment. The freedom to hold hands walking down the street, kiss in public, and cuddle in the hotel bed was magical.

On the last night of their trip. Mara had another first experience with her girlfriend that blew her mind. It started with her lover inserting her fingers inside her. First it was one finger, then two, then three. She continued to work Mara's pussy in a way that she had never experienced before. *What the fuck is happening?* she thought. She eventually came like she never had before, and once her head had cleared, she asked what happened.

"You just got fisted," her girlfriend replied.

The fact that she hadn't even realized what was happening in the throes of their sexual frenzy only added to the hotness of the experience.

As time passed, Mara began to slowly merge her life partners in social settings. Sometimes the three would go to dinner or grab a drink and shoot the shit. Noticing her husband was becoming more comfortable around her girlfriend, Mara decided to revisit the topic of a potential threesome. To Mara's delight her husband was now into it because he had developed a real connection with the girlfriend, and in turn, she also said yes.

At the request of her husband and girlfriend, Mara booked a rental home so the hook up could take place in neutral territory. After dinner the women led Mara's husband into the bedroom where they had a surprise for him. They both dropped their clothes at the same time to reveal the sexy lingerie they had worn just for him. They instructed him to sit in the chair and watch as the two of them climbed onto the bed, got upright on their knees, and started to kiss. Passionate, long, slow, open mouth kisses, while their hands explored each other's bodies. Mara glanced over and saw her husband smiling as he watched the show. Soon, she beckoned him to come join them. He took off his pants and climbed into the bed with them; he was rock hard.

While it was only the second time the girlfriend had been sexually involved with a man, she happily climbed on top to ride him while Mara rode his face. As the orgasms flowed it seemed there were no limits to what they were willing to do with each other. Mara fucked her girlfriend with a strap-on and then watched as her husband fucked her next. Seeing her husband with her girlfriend was icing on the cake. Eight hours later they finally exited the bedroom, thoroughly exhausted.

Not only did the threesome live up to everyone's expectations, it exceeded them. It was absolutely perfect. Everyone's chemistry was on point, and the interactions between the three of them flowed naturally. It was hard to believe how in sync they were. With the threesome a massive success, everyone agreed it should happen again. However, to make sure it wouldn't lose its spark, they decided it would be best to save it for special occasions only.

As the three of them continued to hang out more and more, their connection grew. At first Mara struggled to balance the feelings she had for the both of them. Though her husband was still the love of her life, she had fallen in love with her girlfriend as well. She eventually found that as long as she didn't compare the relationships, she was able to nurture the independent connections she had with each partner.

She has the best of both worlds, a loving husband, and a loving girlfriend, and feels the future is looking incredibly bright for all three of them.

Based on episodes

648 - Mara Got a Free Pass and Is Now In a Poly Relationship with Her Husband and a Woman

731- Mara Has a Husband and a Lesbian Lover and They All Recently Slept Together

CONFESSION XII: MIKE

After his wife left him for a Black bull she had met during one of their swinging and hotwifing experiences, Mike found himself a freshly single fifty-four-year-old bisexual man. Having previously repressed his bisexual side during his marriage, he was finally at a place in his life where he was ready to freely and openly explore it.

Adult Arcades

Mike's first sexual experience, which unexpectedly took place with a male buddy, left a lasting impression on him that shaped his future. Although he knew he was super attracted to women, he was inexplicably drawn to cock too. In between dating girls, he secretly hooked up with guys. Fearing rejection, he kept his bisexual desires a secret. Having no privacy at home and unable to resist the urges, Mike first turned to adult arcades as an escape. The first time he entered one of the private booths, he noticed a button labeled GLASS. He pressed it out of sheer curiosity and when the frosted panel between the neighboring booths turned clear, a man stroking his cock appeared.

"Whoa, wait a minute!" he muttered aloud.

He immediately clicked the button again, to return the privacy shield. With his interest piqued, Mike started frequenting the store once or twice per week. Little by little, as his comfort level increased, he started pressing the GLASS button, jerking off side-by-side with total strangers.

Next Mike started experimenting at adult bookstores. He would go alone and make a beeline for the glory hole booth in the back. Random cock after random cock would push through the hole and Mike sucked them all off. Sometimes Mike wanted a more connected experience, so he wouldn't lock the door hoping someone would come in. Eventually when a guy arrived who wanted to see the action for himself, they would open the unlocked door, and Mike would blow them in the booth. If Mike was lucky, while he was blowing the guy who was in front of him, another guy would push through the glory hole, doubling his fun.

Cruising

Hoping to find more erotic outlets, Mike perused the internet and learned about cruising spots. One night on his way home, he pulled into a known location and witnessed several guys stroking themselves in parked cars. As he walked around checking out the scene, he learned that when he was given "the signal," it was an invitation for him to join in on the fun. Sometimes the participants just watched each other jerk off. Sometimes they stroked each other's cocks. And sometimes they exchanged blow jobs.

He quickly found out that behind the parking lot was a wooded area where more intense hookups went down. Mike saw men constantly entering and exiting the woods. That seemed to be happening whenever Mike went there, at all hours of the night. When he got up the courage to venture beyond the edge of the trees, he found groups of guys fucking and sucking each other. No formal introductions were ever made, and no names were spoken. In the darkness, things escalated quickly for the newbie. First, he was sucking one cock, suddenly there were two, and then there was a line of men waiting.

It was in those woods where Mike got his first spontaneous bottoming experience. While blowing a stranger, the man suddenly spun Mike around, bent him over, spit right on Mike's hole, and pushed his rock-hard dick into his virgin ass. *Oh my God! This is so fucking hot!* he thought to himself. Mike could barely think straight as he grabbed his ankles and took it all in. As he drove home, Mike realized he was totally hooked on the anonymous thrill. He wanted more.

Eventually he stumbled upon bathhouses, which were safer places to fulfill his fantasies. They were equipped with showers, saunas, private rooms, and open public sections with gay porn playing. Throughout the space there were loads of naked men walking around. It was truly a cock lover's paradise.

As an exhibitionist, Mike loved putting on a show. In the dimly lit hallways of the bathhouse, guys would signal they were ready for action by openly jerking off. Mike loved to stroll around, find a guy jerking, and stop to blow him right there in the hallway. He got quite popular and sometimes would remain on his knees surrounded by a group of men watching and waiting for a turn in his mouth.

His Wife and Her Bull

Throughout all these secret explorations, Mike was still dating women, and eventually got married. Over time though, he began to struggle with monogamy and sexual boredom, which resulted in a strain on the marriage. In an effort to spice things up a bit with his wife, he suggested they go to swinger parties together. Moving slowly at first, the couple started as voyeurs before they progressed to soft-swapping and full-swapping. Mike got off watching his wife play with men and women and hoped it would help their relationship get back on track.

One night at a party, Mike and his wife had a threesome with a Black man. He had a monster-sized dick, perhaps the biggest Mike had ever seen. As they played, his wife's mouth bounced back and forth, attending to each of them. When she ended up on the bed, Mike ate her pussy while she continued blowing the well-hung Black man. Everyone was enjoying the hot interaction until Mike looked up and saw his wife kissing the guy, which was against the couple's rules.

As the play continued, Mike backed off a little to watch and was stunned to see the guy fuck her without a condom. Not only was that another violation, but they were not merely fucking—they were passionately making love. His wife was moaning while the guy was slowly moving in and out of her, and sensually kissing her at the same time. *I've never heard her make sounds like that with me*, he thought. His discomfort got worse when she soaked the bed from squirting, another thing he had never seen her do.

On the way home from the party, his wife was elated at the experience. She told Mike she wanted to see the guy again, but next time she wanted to see him alone. Mike was against it, but she went anyway and began to meet up with the bull regularly. Growing uncomfortable with the situation, Mike wanted her to take a break from playing with the guy, but she stubbornly refused. Unable to reach a compromise after several months, they split and eventually divorced. Through the rumor mill, he found out she wound up in a relationship with the bull and they're still together.

Bathhouses

Burying his kinky desires while married had not erased them, and they instantly flooded back with a fierce intensity once he was divorced again. Mike was still attracted to women for a relationship, but the connections he began to seek centered around a thirst for cock. *Lots* of it. The more, the better. So back to the bathhouses he went.

One night, when Mike was on his normal prowl walking down the hall, a muscular Black man stopped him and opened his towel to reveal his BBC. Mike had never been attracted to Black men but when he saw how well-hung that guy was, he became intrigued.

"Wow! What are you going to do with that?" Mike asked.

"I am going to use it on you," the well-endowed gentleman asserted.

Mike grabbed the man's cock, led him into the nearest room, and dropped to his knees. Faced with the biggest dick that he had ever seen, Mike was slightly intimidated. He started to stroke it and rub it all over his face. The man started getting hard and Mike's excitement grew along with it. Although Mike was not exactly sure how long it technically measured, when he jammed it down his throat, he estimated it to be at least eight inches.

Soon Mike was on all fours and the Black stud railed him for nearly half an hour while he pulled his hair and slapped his head. Mike got so hypnotized that he would have done anything he was told to do. *What the fuck was happening?* Mike asked himself. Oddly, while getting pounded, his mind was consumed with flashbacks of his ex-wife. In a bizarre twist, he understood what his wife meant when she said she had never been fucked like that before. Just like her, he was becoming mesmerized by the power of the mighty Black cock.

Trains

Soon after, Mike had his first train experience at a bathhouse. When he peeked into one of the private rooms, he saw two men hooking up and decided to join them. The three of them started running their hands on each other, while stroking each other's cocks, and taking turns on their knees. Soon Mike fell into his submissive role and began alternating his hands and mouth as he serviced the two men. Before he knew it, there was a third man in the room who got behind Mike and started to fuck him.

With one in his hand, one in his mouth, and one in his ass, Mike was very happy being the slutty center of attention. Things only got better when the guy who was fucking Mike finished inside of him and immediately one of the other guys took his place. Soon the second guy came inside him and then the third guy took over. After all three had come inside him, Mike was hooked on trains from that point forward.

Casually falling into a train became routine for Mike. When he popped into the sauna one afternoon, Mike found two guys jerking each other off and figured it was the perfect time to get involved. Offering his open mouth, both eagerly accepted. Soon several more men entered the room and suddenly, Mike was surrounded by six naked men who all took turns on him. God, he truly loved being used!

At one point, while one guy was in his mouth and another guy was behind him, the guy he was blowing suddenly became very aggressive. He grabbed his face and repeatedly pulled his cock out of Mike's mouth to smack him in the face with it. It made him feel like a little bitch, which Mike discovered was a huge turn-on for him. *Pow! Pow! Pow! Damn, that stiff cock was hefty against his cheek*, he thought. One by one the men came all over his face leaving him a dripping, sticky mess. Being left covered in cum from six different guys was the perfect grand finale to the impromptu train.

Discovering His Sissy Side

As time went on, Mike's sissy side started to emerge, and he began attending the cross-dressing themed nights at the bathhouse. He would confidently parade around wearing crotchless panties and thigh-high stockings, waiting to be spanked. Dressing up made it easy for him to fall into the sissy role. On one occasion, Mike was playing on a king-sized bed with one guy and before he knew it, three other guys joined in. Soon, his dainty panties came off and he found himself getting hit from all sides. One guy smacked his ass so hard that he was left sore and welted, but happy, for three days.

Mike thrived on being submissive. The more he played, the more he began to understand that rough treatment and being degraded was a major kink for him. When a man asked him what he was into, Mike often answered, "I want to be your bitch."

When not frequenting bathhouses, Grindr became a useful way for Mike to connect with other partners. With his tagline reading "Cross-dresser seeking guys," each time he logged in, his inbox immediately got flooded with messages. While scrolling through the messages, he struck up a conversation with a hot twenty-two-year-old Black man. The younger guy asked what types of play Mike was into, and Mike explained he was basically a bottom bitch who liked it rough.

As it turned out, the younger guy was a Dom. Realizing they were a good match, Mike reserved a room at the bathhouse for them to meet.

Settling in, Mike unpacked his bag of lingerie and got changed. Soon, the young Dom walked in and dropped his pants.

"Suck my fucking cock!" he demanded.

Whoa! Thought Mike. It was even bigger up close! As Mike blew him, the Black stud forcefully grabbed the back of his head and fucked his face hard. Then, dragging him by the hair, he threw Mike down on the bed and powerfully fucked him for twenty minutes until he exploded in his ass. As the Dom finished his powerful orgasm, he shouted at Mike: "Don't you fucking move!"

Obediently listening to the instruction, Mike lay motionless with the guy's still-hard cock buried in his ass. For nearly ten minutes they stayed that way until the thrusting began again. Rock-hard, he fucked Mike until he came a second time. After finishing, he rolled Mike over and positioned himself directly in front of Mike's mouth.

"Now suck my dick."

Mike orally worked the cock until it erupted a third time. *Holy shit, this guy's stamina was unbelievable,* he thought.

The third time they met, the young Dom was in an extra aggressive mood. He wanted to know how Mike would feel about taking things up a notch. Mike was all in, even though he didn't know what he was agreeing to.

The session started with Mike getting slapped around harder than he had ever been, but he liked it. The guy then grabbed his head and forced his cock so far down Mike's throat that he couldn't even breathe through his nose. The guy then pulled himself out, allowing Mike a quick breath, before he slammed his cock back down his throat. The process repeated itself several times. Mike had never had such a hot experience.

And just when he thought it couldn't get any more intense, the Dom told Mike he was going to fuck him in the ass. As the fucking began, Mike started to grunt and then scream in pleasure/pain. *Holy shit, it hurts so good!* he thought. Even with the guy's hands covering Mike's mouth, his screams could be heard throughout the bathhouse. The noise coming from the private room was so loud that another patron knocked on the door to ensure everything was okay.

"We're fine!" the Dom shouted through the locked door.

Remembering that night still makes Mike laugh.

Trans Girl Threesome

When the Grindr app alerted Mike of a new message, he was thrilled to see who had sent it. The words "Hey, bitch" were from a trans girl he had hooked up with a handful of times. She was with her boyfriend and told Mike they needed some "sissy-pussy" to spice up their evening. The idea of being double-teamed by them was something Mike was definitely up for.

Upon arriving, he was introduced to her slim, smooth boyfriend. He was exactly the type of man Mike was attracted to. In the bedroom, Mike pulled down the guy's pants and was blown away by his gigantic cock.

The couple laid down on the bed and Mike started blowing them both, alternating between the guy's raging nine-inch hard-on and the girl's modest six inches. Then she sat up and started forcing Mike's head further down on her boyfriend's shaft as she shouted at him, "Suck it, bitch! Now suck his fucking balls!"

She and her boyfriend totally ravaged Mike. The boyfriend was the more dominant of the pair, and it seemed like she was submissive to him, but together, they both completely subjugated Mike. They took turns fucking his ass and mouth, using him the way he craved being used. As the couple lay side-by-side on the bed, making out with each other, Mike sucked them off until they came.

But playing with the dominant duo wasn't all just rough and forceful. That night, Mike experienced another first: his first kiss with a guy. Mike was surprised at himself, but also admitted that it felt right and good to him. He enjoyed it so much that he hooked up with the pair three more times.

Mike's adventures frequenting bathhouses, glory holes, and Grindr continues to this day. Sometimes when he reflects on all his debaucherous escapes, even he thinks, *wow, I can't believe I did that.* After decades of salacious adventures, almost entirely with men, the fifty-four-year-old still can't picture himself developing an emotional attachment to a man or having a relationship with one. He really wants that with a woman, and he's hoping to find one who will allow him to continue to play with men. One that he can be up-front with about his sexual identity and kinks. One who will not only allow him to continue to play with men, but will celebrate it. He knows who he is now and can't pretend to be someone he isn't. Meanwhile, Mike continues to have fun with guys, always pushing the boundaries of what he'll do on his crazy adventures.

Based on episodes

580 - Mike Is Secretly into Guys, Glory Holes, Gang Bangs, Swinging, and a Whole Lot More

830 - Mike Is into Glory Holes, Bathhouses, Cross-Dressing, and More

CONFESSION XIII: DAMIEN & RACHEL

When any vanilla couple chooses to enter into the lifestyle, there is always a risk. What if their family members find out, or their neighbors, or in Damien and Rachel's case: what if their religious community found out? Damien and Rachel were practicing members of the Orthodox Jewish community.

Interestingly, when Damien and Rachel married thirty years ago, they were not that religious. But in 2001 they decided to enter into the Jewish community and fully embraced the Orthodox tradition. They kept the Sabbath, abided by Kosher restrictions, and obediently prayed throughout the day. Rachel even stopped wearing pants and began covering her hair and elbows when going out in public; all in accordance with Orthodox Jewish traditions. Not the type to do anything half assed, the couple dove fully into the experience.

Opening Things Up

The devout couple's unexpected journey into the lifestyle started as a simple bucket list joke. Like most guys, Damien fantasized about being with two women. Never expecting a threesome would actually happen, he threw the idea out to Rachel one evening. Humoring her husband, Rachel agreed. They innocently perused hookup apps and commented on which hotties would make a good unicorn for a FMF (female-male-female) threesome. And then one day, out of the blue, the intention shifted from just perusing to reality.

"Why don't we just do it?" Rachel suddenly suggested while scrolling through the array of eligible women.

Damien was surprised, and her suggestion led to a serious discussion about inviting a female into their bedroom. After much debate, Rachel confessed that she would be more comfortable if their first experience was with a guy instead of a girl.

Damien was fine with it. He didn't care how they started, he was just excited to be trying something new. After so many years of monogamous vanilla sex, the thought of anything out of the ordinary was a huge turn-on. But it was Rachel's comment the next morning that really took him by surprise.

"Seeing two guys kissing really turns me on," Rachel blurted out.

She admitted that kissing scenes in gay porn always drove her wild and that the possibility of experiencing it live was exciting. She was curious if her husband would be down to do it. After some thought, he reasoned that since he really wanted to see Rachel make out with another woman it was only fair that she would want the same thing. If she needed this to go down first before she crossed that boundary, he would be a willing participant. He wasn't attracted to men, but it wasn't a deal breaker either. He figured he was just being a good partner.

With their sights set on their first MFM (male-female-male) threesome, they dove into some extensive conversations to make sure they were on the same page. Rachel had genuine concerns.

"What if this screws everything up for us?" she asked.

Damien took his wife's question very seriously. It was a valid worry. They had a good thing going, and they were most definitely taking a risk. But they knew they were a solid team and figured they had a strong enough foundation to deal with whatever came their way. They had navigated many difficult situations during their twenty years of marriage, and they had always come out on top. If this went well, then it would be a great thing they would continue to enjoy. If it all went sideways, then they'd just stop. Open communication would be key, and they decided to move forward and experience their first MFM threesome.

With the decision to go forward, they began searching swinger websites for a man to join them. After a lot of false starts, they found a patient and understanding guy who was looking for a couple to hook up with. His photos were attractive, his demeanor was pleasant, he was okay with the fact that they were newbies, and he was respectful of their boundaries. With all three in agreement, they scheduled a meetup.

When the day finally arrived and they were getting ready in their bedroom together, they both admitted how nervous they were. But they were also both fully committed to giving it a shot. Damien walked over to Rachel, gave her a big, warm hug, and they prepared to take their first step into the wild world of swinging.

Sitting in the cab on their way to the lounge where they planned to meet the mystery man, they sat in silence, holding hands. When they walked in and saw him standing at the bar, a wave of disappointment came over the both of them. It was obvious that the man's photos were from several years prior. But they were so set on going through with it, that they decided to keep an open mind and see where the evening ended up.

They grabbed a booth and initiated an awkward conversation. Neither one of them had any idea how to navigate the situation. It quickly became obvious the man had experience. He was kind and welcoming to all their questions, and they really appreciated how much he put them at ease. After a couple cocktails, they felt more relaxed, and Rachel let Damien know she was into the man. Damien then suggested they move the party back to their place.

After a quick drive back, they walked into the house, took their coats off, and stood there for a moment unsure of what to do next.

Their guest quickly recognized their confusion, took the lead again, and graciously guided them.

With both men knowing what Rachel's desire was, the night started with them gently touching each other. Cognizant of Damien's comfort level as a newbie, the man let him be the one in control of pushing things further.

Rachel was in heaven watching Damien with another man. She couldn't believe it was happening right in front of her. When her husband eventually got on his knees to suck the other man's cock, she nearly exploded. Seeing how turned on she was, the other man returned the favor so she could see Damien getting his cock sucked too. Not wanting to feel left out, Rachel joined in. She started kissing them and stroking their bodies while she watched them orally service one another.

Soon the man asked Rachel if she would like some attention from the men and she nodded yes with a smile. He told her to sit down on the couch, then he kneeled in front of her, spread her legs apart, and went down on her. He was the first man to touch her in that way in twenty years, and it was amazing. Damien sucked on her nipples while the man continued, till Rachel blurred out: "I want to get fucked."

She flipped over so the man, who was already in the correct place, could slip his hard cock right into her ready body. As he grabbed her hips and pushed into her, Damien kissed his wife; he couldn't believe they were really doing it. For the rest of the evening, the two men took turns fucking her and trying several wonderful positions that allowed everyone to be involved.

When they woke up the next morning, the couple couldn't believe they had done it. They had crossed a boundary and were forever changed. And they wanted more. . . . But they did agree that moving forward they should ask for *recent* pictures before meeting someone in person.

Couple Swap

For their next adventure, they decided to try a different dynamic and chose a couple to swap with. They also decided to skip the awkward warm up at the bar, and just invited the couple over to their place. They were an attractive couple and initially they were attentive and engaged.

First, they swapped partners and just kissed, which quickly resulted in clothes peeling off. With everyone naked, touching turned to foreplay and the sounds of oral sex filled the room. When that led to fucking, Damien was finally experiencing his first new woman in twenty years. But just as his excitement and enjoyment was building, Damien and Rachel's dog came into the room and the other woman immediately stopped the sex to play with the dog. Damien wasn't sure what to do as he watched her attention shift completely to his pet. Unfortunately, it continued for the rest of the evening. She was more interested in the dog than Damien, and he was left with no option but to play with Rachel and the other guy.

It was bizarre to say the least and definitely ruined the mood for Damien and Rachel. Somehow, they powered through the strange evening and could say they had their first full couple swap even though it was less than ideal. Later that evening while lying in bed together they contemplated their second experience. It became obvious to the both of them that the perfect scenario was probably going to be hard to find, Damien realized they had two choices and asked Rachel: "Moving forward, do you want to be slutty, or do you want to be selective?"

Rachel laughed. But then quickly got serious and replied: "Let's be slutty."

To her it seemed like it would be a lot more fun to be slutty, and fun was the whole point. She explained her selective phase was when she picked Damien as her husband so many years ago. She was ready for her slutty phase, and Damien gladly agreed.

Exploring Their Slutty Side

The next time they connected with a couple proved to be much more successful. The minute they arrived, everyone was relaxed and in the mood. What started out as touching each other's partners ended up becoming a four-person pile up on their king-sized bed. After an energetic swapping session, while taking a break, Damien decided he wanted to push the fantasy he had really been waiting for.

"Would you like to kiss my wife?" Damien asked.

"I would love to," replied the woman.

Rachel blushed at the woman's response but gave a nod when the woman looked at her for approval. She sat there, heart pounding in her ears as the woman walked over to her, lightly grabbed Rachel's face with her hands, and gently planted a kiss. At the soft touch of the other woman's lips, Rachel melted into the experience and let out a moan.

Damien was on fire. Sitting in a chair, with a glass of whisky in his hand, he watched the women adore each other's bodies. To his amazement, he saw his wife kiss the woman's stomach, and then slide her face down between her wide-open legs to taste her first pussy. Lying flat on the bed, the woman's back was arched up, mouth open, eyes closed, gripping the sheets with both hands, legs trying to spread wider to let Rachel in further. Damien was getting to watch live the porno he had been imagining for years.

In perfect reciprocity, Damien and Rachel both had a bisexual experience, simply because they loved each other enough to provide it.

Keeping within the vibe of trying to please each other by enabling new experiences and fantasies, Damien remembered something that Rachel had once told him. When she was in high school, Rachel had a crush on a Black classmate. Back then interracial relationships were not as accepted as they are now, and the taboo of it only added to her desire. Unfortunately, she never got to experience her fantasy, but she never stopped thinking about it. As far as erotic experiences go, for her, he had been the one that got away. Damien decided to try and find a Black man to finally fulfill Rachel's fantasy.

When he found a guy he thought she'd like, he showed her the photos and she lit up. They started a slow online flirtation over several weeks, taking their time to get to know each other. They talked about sexual likes and dislikes, limits and fetishes, and even exchanged an assortment of X-rated videos to build the tension. By the time he eventually came to their house, the sexual tension was palpable which led to phenomenal sex. Experiencing her first BBC was amazing and he has been a guest in their home several times since. He has even spent the night in their bed, with Rachel sandwiched between both men.

When they met a different Black man who was more open-minded, they were able to push boundaries and officially share him as husband and wife. It was fun to go down on the Black stud together and feel the massive cock inside both their mouths. Each time they hooked up with him, they continued to explore more bi-play. One night, the guy attempted to blow Damien. But after only a few seconds, the guy freaked out and the evening ended. Damien realized the guy-on-guy action might have been too overwhelming because he ghosted them soon after.

Bi-play was still a touchy subject and not all guys were as secure in their identity as Damien was. Damien didn't consider himself bi and would never intentionally seek out another guy, but in the heat of the moment, if a cock was in his face, he had no problem taking it like a champ. Besides, the effect it had on Rachel was priceless. Once the clothes came off, it was common for lines to get blurred. Several men who claimed they were straight had impulsively sucked his cock or jerked him off.

During their sexcapades, they realized that their decision to be slutty sometimes paid off with surprisingly wonderful results. Initially while looking at a particular couple's profile, Rachel didn't find herself attracted to the husband. But the kinky vibe portrayed in their photo gallery instantly drew Damien in. Photos of the wife posed in a ball gag bound with rope and wearing a furry tail were enticing. It seemed most swingers on the site they used offered mainstream vanilla group or swapping sex. It was not common to find members who were heavy into kink and bondage, and therefore it seemed silly to waste the unique opportunity.

Trying Other Things

With Damien intrigued by the bondage and discipline portion of BDSM, he was excited by the possibility of a partner requesting to be tied up. Rachel decided to take a chance on the couple and was pleasantly surprised by the outcome when they all had a great time together. Watching Damien skillfully restrain and spank her impressed Rachel, and she realized it was pretty hot to see him take charge like that. It turned out to be so fun that they played with the couple again.

On another occasion, they tried bringing a male Dom into the bedroom for Rachel's pleasure. She loved it, but Damien was left with an uncomfortable feeling about the whole thing. Damien, who preferred to be the alpha, felt that domming Rachel was *his* role in her life, and was uncomfortable with any other man fulfilling that duty. After crossing that line, they went back to the other side, and to this day, have stayed there.

To branch out, the couple attended a few swinger parties but felt out of place. The environment of spontaneously hooking up with random strangers usually left them playing with each other. Since knowing who they were fucking and building a rapport was crucial for them, club atmospheres didn't particularly suit them. The only small perk the large swinger events provided, however, was it enabled them to fuck in front of other people and feed their exhibitionist appetites.

With numerous scenarios completed, Damien and Rachel fell into a rhythm. Taking it slow and having a contingency plan for everything helped them handle each situation with ease. The ability to adapt and change accordingly also added to their success. Originally, they had superficial rules like not sending red heart emojis to anyone else because that meant love. They only operated with two important guidelines: they always played together in the same room, and both could not be tied up at the same time.

They also realized they preferred group play over separate swaps, especially cuddle puddles. Eventually though, Rachel, who had numerous magical encounters, already felt her experiences in the lifestyle were more plentiful than her husband's. She achieved fucking a BBC, eating pussy, and finding guys she was deeply fond of. In return, she desperately wanted Damien to have even more mind-blowing connections with other women, but it was easier said than done.

Quitting Isn't an Option

Rachel's dive into nonmonogamy wasn't nearly as smooth as Damien's. At fifty-four, she was still untangling years of socialization that told her monogamy was the only blueprint for a relationship and marriage. Rewiring her brain to embrace something different took monumental effort when it came to watching Damien with another woman. Oddly she had no problem with him and another man. In fact, she desired it. This internal conflict, which she fully recognized as hypocritical, created a weird, internal tug-of-war, and occasionally, it got the better of her. More than once, mid-play, Damien would notice her struggling and offer to stop. But to her credit, she always pushed on.

Each time she had a difficult experience they always came out the other side feeling closer because of it. Though Rachel couldn't shake the feeling that she needed to get past her issues. Damien, always thinking of her first, suggested several times that they could quit swinging altogether. But Rachel's response was always the same: "No way."

Quitting wasn't in her DNA. She never backed out just because something was hard. She threw herself into everything she did, and this was no different. So, instead of walking away, she decided to push herself further. She devoured every book she could find, listened to podcasts on compersion, and vowed to figure it all out. It was her next challenge, and Rachel wasn't about to give up.

She even got the phrase "I can stand it" tattooed on her wrist as a reminder of her inner strength. *I know he loves me. I can do this. He's not going home with her, this is just fun*, became her mantra. When her husband complimented another woman on her looks or sexiness, she reminded herself that it didn't change the way he felt about her. In what most would consider a short period of time, she has come a long way. Although she still doesn't enjoy watching him with other women, she can deal with it, which is most definitely a step in the direction she wants to go.

Unlike Rachel, jealousy is never an issue for fifty-two-year-old Damien. Rachel is his favorite porn star. *She's hot and she's mine,* he always says to himself. No matter who she fucks, she's going home with him. As long as she was having fun, he was happy. For him, the only negative part of the whole endeavor was seeing the emotional struggle his wife was going through at times.

But other than Rachel's ongoing emotional journey, the two of them have found pleasure in behaving like a pair of rowdy Amish teenagers during Rumspringa. The feeding frenzy continues as they have now met over a dozen men, women, and couples. Between new partners and repeat playmates, they usually swing once or twice a week. And in addition to accomplishing a slew of sexual fantasies in less than a year, Rachel also got her nipples and clitoris pierced.

While they acknowledge they are undoubtedly misbehaving as far as their religious community is concerned, they are very clear that they are not condoning their actions or attempting to persuade others to follow. Beyond a few close friends that know, they are constantly managing the secret to make sure their kids, or the greater Jewish community, doesn't find out. They know that if it ever became public, it would probably result in them being shunned and excommunicated. Damien and Rachel agree that the two conflicting sets of values can't coexist forever. One weekend night they are celebrating the Sabbath with their community and children, the next night they are having a wild foursome. But they both agree that life is for living. So, for now, they are searching for a happy medium between where they have been for most of their lives, and where they seem to be going for the rest of it.

Based on episode

439 - Damien and Rachel were Super Religious' and They're Now In the Lifestyle

CONFESSION XIV: EVE

Eve is a highly sexual cuckquean whose greatest thrill is watching her husband fuck other women, leaving Eve to clean up the mess. But she didn't start out that way. Her journey from the highly repressed religious community she grew up in, to being the matriarch of a "Fuckhouse on the Hill," was a wild one.

Eve is from a small town in the deep South and grew up in a religious household. In that environment, the female body was so stigmatized that when she got her first period she had no idea what it was. Sexuality was treated as though it didn't exist. They never talked about sex and she had no idea about the mechanics of it. The only thing that she and the other women in her community were taught was not to give away their "forbidden fruit" until they were married.

As Eve entered her teenage years, she began to sense that she was different. She realized she was more attracted to women than to men, but experimenting with anyone, especially women, wasn't really an option in her hometown.

So after getting a boyfriend in her mid-teens, they started having sex, and Eve wound up pregnant. Being extreme religious conservatives, her parents forced her to get married, and by the time she graduated high school, she was living with her husband and baby. Like most marriages of very young couples, life together was confusing and complicated. It didn't help that when Eve confided in her husband about her attraction to women, he shamed her for it. They ended up getting divorced after only a couple years.

Overcoming Repression

Newly single and having repressed a large part of her sexuality up to that point, Eve decided that she wanted to finally explore her attraction to women. As she walked into a bar one evening, Eve noticed a slightly older woman in a pencil skirt sitting alone. As they talked over drinks, the conversation quickly turned flirtatious. The attractive woman leaned over and seductively asked Eve if she wanted to have a drink with her up in her room. Eve eagerly accepted the invite.

As they rode up in the elevator, the two couldn't keep their hands off each other. When the doors opened onto the third floor, they practically stumbled into the hallway with their lips locked. Once in the room, Eve took control of the situation and guided the woman to sit on the edge of the bed. When she saw the woman was not wearing any panties, Eve just went for it and started going down on her.

"Damn, you taste delicious."

Eve looked up to see the woman's head tilt back in ecstasy as her hips pressed her body closer to Eve's mouth. Eve continued to go down on her for the next forty-five minutes. Unfortunately, the night ended earlier than Eve would have liked because the woman's husband walked in on them and tried to join in. Eve had no interest in a threesome, so she left. After getting her first taste of someone else's forbidden fruit, Eve was hooked and couldn't wait to have more.

Growing tired of the suffocating religious environment that she was, out of habit, still a part of, Eve decided to abandon her faith in search of more open-minded options. A fellow mother at her child's school suggested she check out the pagan community that she was part of. She described it as "wonderfully accepting of everybody."

Intrigued, Eve visited the community and was welcomed with friendly, open arms. As a young, attractive horny woman she became quite popular in a free-spirited, free love community.

Becoming a Unicorn

One night after the pagan Christmas party, she was invited back to the house of a couple she had recently become friendly with. As soon as she arrived, they all settled into the living room, and the couple started to make out on the couch. Eve got turned on as she watched from across the room. She felt awkward but also quite aroused, and hoped the couple would invite her to join. Mostly because she was very attracted to the wife and wanted to play with her.

Soon the woman had her husband's pants open and was gently stroking him. She motioned for Eve to come over. As soon as Eve was within reach, the woman gently took her hand, and placed it on her husband's cock. Eve, who really appreciated being told what to do, gladly followed her lead.

After several minutes of stroking the husband, he was rock hard, at which point he instructed Eve to taste his wife. Eve slid over to face the woman, who pulled her panties to the side, and then Eve obediently buried her face in between the woman's thighs. With Eve on her knees and her ass in the air, the husband got behind her, lifted her skirt, and slid his cock inside of her. She was in heaven.

The woman moaned uncontrollably and urged Eve to slide two fingers inside her while the man had his hands on Eve's hips, moving in and out of her. The couple worked Eve in perfect unison and the threesome finished with everyone orgasming simultaneously. From that point on, Eve became obsessed with the thrill of being the unicorn in an MFF (male-female-female) threesome. It also seemed like an easy way to get access to lots of women and that was exactly what Eve was primarily looking for.

The pagan couple had heavy ties in the swinger community and Eve soon found herself at her first swinger house party. She was a huge hit. Word had spread that Eve was down to hook up with couples, and many sought her out.

Eventually Eve started exploring outside of the pagan community, and started frequenting local swingers' clubs. She went there looking for hot couples who were interested in having a female join them and she never had a problem finding those who were down. She was in such high demand that she rarely hooked up with the same couple twice. Most of the time she never even exchanged names or numbers with the couples because she always knew she could find more.

When it came to women, Eve had a weakness for thick, curvy, big-breasted ladies with fat asses. As for men, her tastes were more versatile since she regarded them as spare parts in the scene, considering them a necessary obstacle between her and the women she really wanted to be with. Kissing was very intimate to her, and while she loved kissing women, she had no interest in touching a guy's lips. She had no problem playing with their cocks though if the situation warranted it.

After a couple years of running wild as a unicorn in the pagan community, Eve decided it was time to move on. Soon after, she met a cute guy at a party who caught her attention. Even though Eve was not really into guys, she became enamored with his ability to make her laugh from within her belly and started having regular sex with him. As they continued to get to know each other in and out of the bedroom, Eve started to develop a deep connection to him. They moved in together a few months later, and eventually they married.

Soon Eve's desire for women started bubbling up again, and she asked her husband how he would feel about another woman joining them in bed. Unfortunately, he was not so keen on the idea. He explained that he and his ex had tried opening their relationship a few times, but it had always ended up in a trainwreck. Though his ex always said she was cool with it, whenever it was his turn to hook up or swap, she immediately got filled with jealousy and it tore them apart. Eve assured him that she was not like his ex and swore she would never get jealous. He didn't believe her and shut it down. But Eve would not be dissuaded from getting what she wanted and hatched a plan to convince him.

Surprise Threesome

She decided to set up a surprise threesome for him with a female coworker with whom she was super close. Eve had previously disclosed her wild threesomes to her and she noticed the woman always seemed aroused by the stories. Conveniently for Eve, the coworker had just broken up with her boyfriend. So a week after the conversation with her husband, Eve proposed sharing her husband with her. The coworker immediately jumped on the plan.

The following night, Eve's husband returned home from work to a sexy surprise. As he entered the house, he saw Eve standing in the doorway of their bedroom, wearing a robe, beckoning him to come in. As soon as he stepped foot in the room, he saw her coworker lying on the bed naked. Eve dropped her robe to the floor and jumped onto the bed to join her.

Her husband was in shock and remained frozen in the doorway as he tried to analyze the situation. Eve and her friend started touching each other as her husband continued to stare at the women. Finally, Eve blurted out: "Well if you're not going to eat her pussy, then I will."

With her coworker lying naked on her back, Eve got into position above her, kept her eyes locked on her husband's, and sensually licked her friend's stomach down toward her slowly spreading legs. As she writhed around from Eve's attention, the coworker invited Eve's husband to take his clothes off and join them. After several minutes of watching his wife go down on her, he was finally convinced that the invitation was genuine. He peeled his clothes off and jumped in.

Eve took control and directed all of the activities as the three of them went at it all night long. It was the first time she had a threesome with a man she was emotionally involved with, and watching him with another woman was the biggest turn-on. It was an entirely new feeling for her. She couldn't believe how much she loved it.

Becoming a Cuckquean

After that first experience Eve quickly set up another one with her friend Mary. Mary was a beautiful woman who she had been lusting after for months. When Eve brought her over, Eve's husband was completely on board. Eve sat back and smoked a blunt in a chair as she enjoyed the show that was taking place on their bed. As her husband was on his knees with his face buried between Mary's legs, Eve thought to herself, *My god, I love watching him eat pussy.* Insanely turned on, Eve directed the hot action. When her husband moved in to fuck Mary from behind, Eve interjected with a better idea.

"No, get on top of her."

Eve thought her husband deserved to see her beautiful breasts while he fucked her. Eve climbed on the bed next to Mary so she could also get a good view of the action. Occasionally her husband kissed Eve as he fucked Mary, or Eve kissed her as she fondled Mary's beautiful breasts. Mostly, she just loved watching her husband fuck Mary.

From then on, Eve was on a mission to share her husband. The pleasure of watching him was the high she continually chased. She did have one boundary though, he couldn't come while fucking another woman in the missionary position. Eve didn't want her man looking at another woman when he orgasmed, because she felt that that was a privilege only she deserved to enjoy. What she really loved though, was having him gaze into *her* eyes and describe how amazing and wet their guests felt as he finished inside of them.

Eve's evolution continued when they had a young woman rent a room in their big house. Eve was attracted to her from the get-go, and soon they were all hooking up, and living together. Anything went—sometimes all three were involved, sometimes just the women played, and sometimes just her husband and the roommate fucked. Eve was officially in a throuple, with no hierarchy or jealousy, and she loved it.

Eve was so hooked on watching her husband with other women that she frequently hosted naked rendezvous for her girlfriends at their big house. She would invite them over to do silly craft projects like butt canvases. By the end of the evening, they were all running around the house naked covered in paint, and decorating big white boards with their naughty body parts.

Eve's husband was always nominated to clean their paint covered bodies and from there the sexcapades began. On one particular night with four women over, they took turns fucking each other with a strap on. Eventually, Eve's friends begged for a real cock and her husband was finally allowed to join in.

Round and round they went taking turns with the strap on and the real cock. As one of her girlfriends sucked her husband's cock, another sat on his face, while the third rode a big dildo that he held upright with his free hand. As Eve sat back and took in the whole scene, she realized watching her husband with multiple women was what she loved the most. After he finished inside all of them, she proceeded to clean her husband's cum out of each and every one of them.

After seeing her husband with a ton of women, she realized she was a full-fledged cuckquean and began to encourage her husband to go out and hook up solo. But he wasn't interested. He preferred to play with other women when she was around. And as much as she wanted her husband to play with other women, she couldn't imagine playing with any other man. She only wanted him. She swore if anything ever happened to her husband she would be done with dick forever.

Eve's most recent adventure was the craziest one yet and involved her husband's ex. She was the mother of his child and when she needed a place to stay, Eve suggested she move in. She thought, *maybe a little healthy competition would motivate her to up her own game and become a better wife.* And she was hoping one day they would all fuck . . .

Even though Eve is very happy with her open marriage, she has to contend with a lot of negative judgment from those around her. Besides recently dealing with the judgment from her friends for letting her husband's ex move in, she continues to deal with the backlash for sharing her husband, as well as for hosting swinger parties at their house. The locals have nicknamed her house "The Fuck House" and word on the street is that if you're a guest at their house, you wind up naked and become a notch on Eve's belt.

Regardless, now, at thirty-three, Eve feels very grounded in who she is and she's more secure in her marriage than she has ever been. Though she respects the fact that some people want to be monogamous, she doesn't understand why she can't get the same respect back. That's all she's ever really wanted: to be respected for exactly who she is. But Eve knows she's stronger than the haters, and after doing so much work on herself, she's proud of her journey and where she has arrived. Living according to the adage "To Each Their Own" is her guiding principle, with no plans to change anytime soon.

Based on episode

737 - Eve Is a Bisexual Cuckquean Who Loves Watching Her Husband with Other Women

CONFESSION XV: CRIMSON

They say you shouldn't mix business with pleasure, but Crimson, a former nurse, couldn't disagree more. That's why at sixty-seven, the free-spirited grandmother joined the lifestyle and became a porn star.

Throughout her life, when it came to watching porn, Crimson didn't want to be distracted by unnecessary storylines and cheesy plots. She had a habit of anxiously fast-forwarding to the juicy graphic parts, since the hardcore fucking and penetration were all she needed to see. If she could orgasm in five minutes or less from the steamy scenes, then she was happy. Unfortunately, controlling the pleasure in her real life was a little more complicated.

Throughout her dating history, she always had a higher sex drive than her partners. She constantly felt like a chameleon, having to tone her personality down and adapt to what her partner expected. During her thirty-year monogamous marriage, the sex dwindled until it became completely nonexistent. The lack of passion and intimacy left Crimson discontented and restless. After she divorced her husband at sixty-five, she found herself free to begin exploring her sexuality. It was a world that she had been absent from for so long.

Her First Lifestyle Cruise

Crimson soon discovered the enticing world of swinging. In Southeast Florida where she lived, the scene was prolific, and she rejoiced in the freedom to express herself. Due to her high energy levels and zest for life, Crimson was known to jump into things with both feet. That was evidenced by her first lifestyle event being a seven-day Bliss Cruise she attended alongside 3,500 other swingers.

Right after boarding the massive ship, the first thing she and her date saw was a marvelous ten-couple orgy. For the entire week, the atmosphere was nonstop sex and wild partying. Hookups were constantly taking place in staterooms, plus the numerous indoor and outdoor playrooms. Once at sea, guests could be naked at the pool in addition to several other areas of the vessel. Although patrons were not supposed to be nude in the hallways, the definition of "naked" was very different from what vanilla people would expect. When Crimson wore a see-through mesh top or full body paint with no actual clothing to formal dinners, she was technically considered "dressed."

Crimson was having a blast, but unfortunately, her travel partner was not as into the vibe as she was. After some pressing, he explained his previous vacation partners were vanilla women, and he wasn't prepared for Crimson to actively partake in the kinky festivities. She told him his presumptions had been foolish.

Regardless of his insecurities, she was determined to have a fabulous time even if it meant partying solo. Crimson embraced every moment and viewed it as an opportunity to expand her horizons, discovering what she liked or didn't like. It also allowed her to see all the various sexual activities that people were into. Whether or not she understood why, she appreciated the uniqueness.

While on board, the social butterfly met a charming OBGYN and his wife. They had been married for forty years when they ventured into the lifestyle as a way to freshen up their boring sex life. They were kind enough to educate Crimson about swinging and happy to play a supporting role on her liberating journey.

After she returned from the trip, Crimson received a generous invitation from them. They wanted her to visit them for the holidays so they could teach her more about the lifestyle. The doctor and his wife promised it would be worth the trip.

Always up for an adventure, Crimson flew to Kansas City the day after Christmas and spent nine fabulous days with them. Seven of those nights, they hosted epic house parties in the addition that was built specifically for sex. She was mesmerized by the area containing a four-person shower, a large hot tub, a bed, and a cable restraint system suspended from the ceiling. As the newest member of the social circle, which consisted of all couples, the single Crimson received a lot of flattering attention. She bonded with one of the wives who happened to be a nurse as well.

Heavy into BDSM, the new friend and her husband performed a dramatic scene that Crimson watched with wide-eyed fascination. The wife's hands were secured to a chain hanging from the ceiling and a blindfold was covering her eyes. She was at her husband's mercy. First, he gave her ass a few spanks with his palm to warm her up. Then he skillfully used a leather paddle to increase the intensity and impact. Each time the paddle made contact, her body writhed. Her high-pitched moans were a combination of pleasure and pain as her skin turned pink and welted. After the scene ended, they tenderly kissed. Crimson felt she could truly sense the love between them.

When Crimson got back home, she created a profile on a swinger's dating site to make more connections and was blown away by the number of people that seemed to be enchanted by her. She received message after message from a wide variety of suitors. The GILF was a hot commodity, and sometimes four or five hundred messages a week filled her inbox. Living it up, Crimson fucked a lot and didn't mind when playmates filmed the intimate dates or took souvenir photos.

Going Pro

She realized that if videos and photos were already being taken during her dates, she might as well monetize off of them. If she could have fun doing that and make money at the same time, she considered it to be a dream come true.

An enlightening conversation with a twenty-year-old college student she was banging guided her further in the right direction. The young man, who was forty-six years her junior, told her about a website called SexyJobs where people posted all types of stuff about the adult industry.

"I bet you could make a lot of money," the young hottie informed her.

Having recently left her prestigious job in healthcare, Crimson had blown through her savings and needed income, so she figured she might as well try something adventurous. She contemplated if establishing herself in the adult industry as a sixty-seven-year-old grandmother was realistic or just a far-fetched fantasy.

With nothing to lose, Crimson searched the website designed to help producers and talent meet. Once she created a profile, messages from several people offering gigs immediately piled up. Based on intuition, she chose a company in Tampa called Private Society. It was owned by a married couple, and Crimson liked the fact that they had turned their house into a film studio. When she showed up for her first job, she was told it was an unscripted scene because the director wanted the sex to occur naturally between them. She sat and chatted with the other actor for a bit to break the ice before filming, so she could at least have some sort of connection with him.

The shoot went great, and after she got paid for the sex she had on camera, she realized she was officially a porn star. She smiled to herself as she thought about it, since it had been such an unlikely path. Raised in a conservative household where she never felt good enough, Crimson struggled with self-esteem for most of her life. Twenty-five years ago, she was quite heavy and suffered from body issues before losing over two hundred pounds through diet and exercise. She had been coming out of her repressed shell for the last few years and in her new profession, she found the success and recognition she had been yearning for her whole life. Even though the company in Tampa hardly paid anything, Crimson continued to work with them because she genuinely liked it. In addition, she developed connections with other studios ranging from amateur to professional.

Crimson did initially worry what would happen if her children and grandchildren discovered her sexy new career. But she decided the risk was minimal since they all lived in Europe. Also, since sex had become such a big part of her life since her divorce, she thought if they found out, so be it. Identifying as a sexual renegade after harboring so much guilt for so long, the vivacious GILF was finally ready to live her life unapologetically.

Threesomes, Foursomes, and Moresomes

As a sexual dynamo, Crimson often played with multiple men to maintain a longer-lasting supply of functioning equipment. Although she did occasionally have one-on-one encounters, Crimson truly preferred MFM (male-female-male) threesomes after discovering how much she loved double penetration. Kyle, a lifestyle friend who enjoyed pleasuring women, (previously mentioned in Confession IX) helped arrange groups for her. As an older man with a huge cock that didn't always cooperate, it was his way of being able to still give her pleasure. Generally, four men created the perfect balance for her. When the first two were exhausted, the remaining two could rotate in to give the first pair of suitors time to recover for the next round.

It's interesting to note that Crimson considered this type of arrangement, a MMFMM, (male-male-female-male-male) merely a hookup. For her to consider it a legitimate gang bang, more guests were required. At that point in her journey, her largest gang bang included ten people, but she had hopes to increase that number in the future. Someone did once ask her to fuck one hundred and seventy-six guys in a single night to break the existing record, but she decided that was not something she wanted to be known for.

Thriving and Being Appreciated

Whether it was getting the ball rolling at a swinger event or starting a spontaneous orgy, Crimson was the life of the party and people gravitated toward the carefree type of environment she created. During one event, Crimson found herself to be the center of attention in a playroom during a massive gang bang. When the area got closed, they had to find a new location to continue the fun. As she walked through the lobby hallway, everyone at the bar watched as five guys trailed Crimson, making her feel like the Pied Piper.

As an older woman, people were often surprised by Crimson's impressive sexual appetite. She turned to bioidentical hormone replacement pellets to keep her body regulated. So far, it has worked like magic as she could still spend an entire weekend fucking and be fine. Blessed with a high libido and energy to match, she considered herself a medical anomaly since the years have not slowed her down at all.

One thing that she really appreciated was how the adult industry recognized that older people were sexual creatures and represented them more and more in content. Although there was still negativity regarding sex and aging women, many men legitimately preferred older lovers. Crimson was happy to be proof that women could be horny sex symbols at any age.

Since her divorce, Crimson sporadically dated, but guys often wanted her to leave the lifestyle or the adult industry, both of which she refused to do. Staying positive, she cautiously waited to see how each new relationship unfolded since it was common for men to draw the line at women earning money for sex. To any man uncomfortable with her empowered attitude, she always gave them the same response: "I finally feel like I am part of a group, and I am not leaving it for anyone."

She told them they could either join her for the journey, or she would gladly travel alone.

When Private Society hosted a special event in Iowa where subscribers could meet the talent, Crimson got the thrill of a lifetime. The sexual tension in the room was thick as four female starlets and one male performer mingled with fans. One by one, participants undressed until everyone was naked. With the stars leading the way, an orgy which involved seven women and over forty guys getting down and dirty for three hours ensued. During the marathon of sex, with random body parts constantly entering all parts of her, Crimson lost track of how many guys she hooked up with. Aside from being tangled in the pile of dozens of random limbs, her favorite part was the fact that she outlasted all the younger women. As usual, insatiable Crimson was the last woman standing.

In Sickness and in Health

But right when Crimson was on top of the world with her new life, she was hit with a double diagnosis of breast cancer and coronary heart disease. Surgery was necessary for both. As she lay in the hospital bed the night before the open-heart surgery, a male friend came by to keep her company. As he sat in a chair across the room from her bed, images of his familiar hard cock fluttered through her mind while they chatted about mundane things. As her mind wandered, and memories of the countless times he had exploded in her mouth came up, she decided she needed to suck his cock right then and there. Hell, it might be the last cock she ever got to suck, she reasoned. When she told him what she wanted to do, he was shocked and called her crazy for suggesting it. He was certain they would get caught. But his concerns did not dissuade the horny patient.

She hopped out of bed and placed a pillow on the floor to kneel right in front of his chair. As she unzipped his pants, Crimson remained focused as she released him from his boxers. Her mouth watered at the sight of his magnificent cock only a few inches away from her face. As she teased him with his jeans crumpled around his ankles, she could sense him tense up each time they heard muffled voices or footsteps in the hallway.

But his fears seemed to melt away as she wrapped her hungry lips around him and proceeded to slide all the way down. He felt heavenly in her mouth, and she loved how he grew harder each time the tip hit the back of her throat. He bit his lip, closed his eyes, and tried not to moan too loudly from her exceptional oral skills. Given that it was still before midnight when he came in her mouth, she figured swallowing it would be the perfect pre-surgery protein boost.

The triple bypass surgery she underwent the next day required Crimson to be hospitalized for a week and unfortunately, she contracted a very serious case of Covid-19 during her stay. Even though she had barely begun her recovery from the open-heart surgery, she was forced to undergo not one, but *two* lung surgeries. The five-week period of multiple procedures took a heavy toll on her body.

For the first month of her being home, Crimson barely did anything other than sleep all day and all night. Her body was so weak that even small tasks like going downstairs or eating were too strenuous. Being confined to her bed was lonely for the party animal, but thankfully many friends stayed in touch, which lifted her spirits a bit.

By week six of being confined to her house, two male friends were especially concerned by her mood, so they arranged to visit one Friday night. For the next forty-eight hours, the three pals partied without a care in the world. It was nice to enjoy each man's body without rushing. Sometimes she played with one while the other watched and other times she had both on her simultaneously. She orgasmed like crazy in all the wonderful positions they could manage with her weakened body. In between rounds they laughed, ate snacks, and genuinely enjoyed hanging out with each other.

Reconnecting with her wild side was therapeutic for Crimson's mental health and physical well-being. The erotic hangout was so fabulously wonderful that they did it again the following weekend. Crimson truly believed the endorphins released from the sex were responsible for jump-starting her recovery. The powerful orgasms awakened her and motivated her to continue to work hard to regain her strength. A few weeks later, at a follow-up appointment with her doctor, she was informed that she could return to her normal activities. Crimson just smiled and thought to herself, *Well, I already have been.* (Please note that you should always consult your doctor after any medical procedure as to when it is safe for you to resume regular activities, including anything sexual.)

Crimson wasted no time jumping back into her thriving social life. The first event she attended was a lifestyle New Year's Eve party in Orlando in honor of hotwives and women who love Black men. Being immersed in a room full of people fucking and fooling around was thrilling, strutting around in lingerie again was refreshing.

Back in Action

Three months later, Crimson was in full make-up-for-lost-time mode when she attended a hotel takeover. At about 1:30 a.m., she casually strolled down the halls, scoping out the scene in each playroom. She was trying to find an exciting group she could join when she met a man who invited her to play. They soon found an empty room and jumped on each other. While on her hands and knees with her back to the door, she could hear other people coming in to watch. Crimson wasn't bothered by the growing crowd; she loved the attention.

Soon though, some of the viewers decided watching wasn't enough. Suddenly, there was a new cock in front of her, and she eagerly took it into her mouth. Then there was another, and another, and another. Before long, the equal opportunity GILF was in the middle of a swarm of drooling men, each awaiting their turn with her.

The festivities were supposed to end at 3 a.m., but with so many still wanting her attention, the security guards allowed the show to go on. After all, they were enjoying the raunchy display as well. Bystanders cheered and applauded as she serviced each stiff cock. By the time the gang bang ended at 4 a.m., Crimson estimated she fucked at least twenty-five guys. She was thrilled to know that each man was going to bed utterly satisfied, but she was not tired yet.

As the crowd dispersed, Crimson noticed one man stayed behind. She realized he had tried to fuck her earlier but had erection issues due to the pressure of being watched. He was shy but sweet, and as they chatted, Crimson felt connected to him in some way. With more energy to spare, she ended up going home with him, and they fucked until 7 a.m. The chemistry was so sublime that they hooked up several nights in a row and an incredibly lovely friendship began to blossom.

At another swinger party in Kansas City, Crimson ventured into sensory deprivation. Placed on a massage table in a conference room, her legs were spread, and her ankles were snugly bound. Someone slipped a satin blindfold over her eyes while someone else inserted earplugs. She writhed in ecstasy as anonymous hands and mouths repeatedly teased her vulnerable body. She felt fingers slide inside her pussy while another set of hands fondled her tits. Her nipples hardened and her thighs trembled as she wondered who was doing what. Unable to see or hear what was happening to her made the experience extremely erotic. It was simply another amazing moment to add to her list.

Five months after her traumatic medical ordeal, Crimson was happier than ever. From overcoming societal judgment, self-esteem issues, insecure partners, menopause, cancer, heart surgery, and much more, the bold GILF continued to attack life to the fullest with absolutely no regrets. She loves sex and feels no shame for it. She felt that coming to terms with her sexuality not only helped her self-esteem but also changed her life for the better in countless ways.

Based on episodes

554 - Crimson Recently Became a GILF Porn Star and Swinger
877 - Crimson Is into Gang Bangs, Black Men, Lifestyle Events, and More
Her OnlyFans: https://onlyfans.com/crimsongilf69

CONFESSION XVI: CRAIG

Craig could never have anticipated the peculiar twist his life would take after his girlfriend of two years dumped him for the class bully. With each passing day, what started as a painfully humiliating situation morphed into an erotic, lifelong cuckolding obsession.

He was crushed by the breakup and having to constantly watch his ex-lover kiss someone else was brutal to endure. Knowing his classmates pitied him only added to his despair. However, the more he thought about his ex-girlfriend with her new boy, the more aroused he got. His body's reaction left him utterly dumbfounded. It got so intense, when he saw them together he frequently had to run home to release his uncontrollable desire. As he lay there in his room stroking himself, he would think about their naked bodies grinding together, and it drove him wild. When he briefly got back together with her, every time they had sex, he pictured her with the other guy. Each time he imagined her coming at the hands of the man who stole her from him, he erupted in uncontrollable orgasms.

His Girlfriend and Her Boss

Craig joined the army at eighteen. Being a young, strong, good-looking man in uniform, he soon got together with a very sexy young woman. The girl was an attractive office worker at a logistics company whose spectacular tits garnished a lot of attention everywhere she went, including at the office. It was all in good fun, and the innocent flirtatious interactions from her coworkers did not initially cause Craig to react.

One evening though, she returned home and groaned about her boss's annoying antics. The innocent flirtations had started to cross the line and he had begun to get very touchy-feely with her. She complained that she constantly caught him staring at her legs and her ass. When Craig heard this, all the vivid memories of his high school arousals rushed back in and filled his mind with new tantalizing ideas. *Was it possible to recapture those emotions with someone else?* he wondered. It was too tempting not to try. Craig tested the waters and encouraged his girlfriend to tease the forty-year-old man.

He suggested she should accidentally let her skirt ride up so he could catch a glimpse, and to wear a low-cut shirt that would accentuate her cleavage. His girlfriend shrugged it off as a stupid joke, but the next morning, Craig selected an outfit for her to wear to work—stockings, a short skirt, and a silk blouse that could easily be unbuttoned.

"Are you fucking nuts, he'll be all over me?" she laughed.

He assured her he was serious and told her to just go for it if he wanted more than just a feel. She was slightly confused but willing to play along. She put on the outfit, and headed to the office. Later that day, after leaving a client's location with her boss, the two were in the company car ready to drive back when the boss took the tempting bait. Daringly, he reached out and ran his hand up her smooth leg. Just as she was about to swat his hand away, she paused as she replayed her conversation with Craig that morning.

The boss took her silence as a signal to keep going. Instead of objecting as she normally would have, she decided it was the perfect opportunity to find out how Craig would really feel if she let her boss fully cross the line. She had to admit, she did find him quite attractive, and after a short internal debate, her thighs slowly spread open to invite his fingers inside. His touch made her body tremble, and she sank deeper into the seat to allow his hand to reach further inside her. She moaned in delight and bit her lower lip as her juices soaked his fingers. She was extremely turned on and decided to do something even bolder. Caught up in the moment, she leaned over, unbuckled his belt, took his cock out, and slid him into her mouth. The boss was so aroused by his stunningly hot twenty-something-year-old employee sliding her mouth up and down on him, that he came within a minute. Afterward, she bashfully wiped her mouth and straightened her clothes and prayed she had understood Craig correctly.

Upon returning home, she hesitantly confessed her dirty deed. Not only was Craig not angry, he was so insanely aroused that he immediately took her right there on the floor of the living room while she described the racy encounter. Hearing the juicy details about how she sucked his cock and how wet it made her, drove him wild. With his encouragement, the blow jobs continued regularly before the boss finally invited her to a hotel room to take the hookup to the next level. By then, she didn't even think twice about satisfying her urges. She reported the details over the phone to Craig while he was away on a training mission. She could hear his powerful orgasm erupt right as she described her own orgasm from being fucked on the bed face down by her boss. Both seemed to enjoy the unconventional direction their relationship was taking. A few months later, they married.

The military base Craig was stationed at frequently sponsored exchange programs among the European forces and Craig's unit hosted the Dutch commandos. One night while they were all out at a nightclub, one of the Dutchmen made quite an impression on Craig's bride so they invited him back to the married quarters to continue the party privately.

Craig sat in a chair while he watched the handsome Dutch officer slow dance with his wife right in front of him. While the officer started kissing her and removing her shirt, Craig practically vibrated out of his chair. Hearing his wife tell stories of her trysts was one thing, but getting a live show aroused the fuck out of him. He watched the handsome man unclip her bra and take her huge bare breasts into his hands. He marveled at his young beautiful wife, who removed her skirt and got down on her knees to take the officer's pants off. He watched as the officer picked her up and laid her on the couch. And finally, he watched as the Dutch officer climbed onto her and slid his big beautiful cock inside her. It was apparent that Craig had crossed the line into full cuckoldry.

Naughty games were easy and natural with his first wife, both being young and carefree. But like many marriages between very young people, as they grew up, they grew apart, and eventually divorced. Craig wondered if he would ever be able to find another woman who would be willing to fulfill his cuckolding desires.

The New Hotwife

A couple years later he met his soon-to-be wife Jane and was instantly taken with her. As they got to know each other and started dating, he occasionally would weave in questions about her ex-boyfriends. He wanted to know how many sexual partners she had and what crazy things she had done. Occasionally when she was receptive to his inquiries, he would probe deeper. He wanted more details.

Jane revealed that when she was twenty-two and her long-term boyfriend had broken up with her, she went out and slept with three of his friends as revenge. She admitted that act had awakened something inside her and she went on a sexual exploration spree. One thing in particular that she found out she enjoyed was hooking up with attached men. She was thrilled at the thought of being impossible to resist. Other times, she and her girlfriends had same-room sex with guys they met on vacation.

As he heard more, he grew increasingly curious about the physical features of her partners and pushed her for further details. The cuck inside him was hoping to hear that their cocks were bigger and better than his, but Jane was reluctant to answer. With time and patience though, he eventually convinced her to open up and was pleasantly shocked by her admission. It turned out, Jane had enjoyed a plethora of well-hung lovers throughout the years.

Craig loved learning about his wife-to-be's wild side. After he gave her an in-depth explanation of his mental draw to cuckolding, he encouraged her to fulfill her fantasies. Jane's interest was certainly piqued when she understood that she could still have novel sexual experiences even though she was married. She quickly embraced the unique position to reap the benefits of two worlds—the security of an adoring loyal husband and the freedom to enjoy unrestricted sexual bliss.

As they embarked on their hotwife journey, one of his favorite memories occurred during a week-long off-site work conference that she attended at a nearby hotel. Craig desperately wanted her to sleep with one of the managers who was always hitting on her, and pushed her to make it happen at the off-site. Much to his delight she agreed and got way more than either of them expected.

While Jane flirted with the manager as planned, she noticed two army men kept staring at her from across the bar. When the crowd died down and coworkers dispersed, one officer covertly slipped Jane a piece of paper with a room number and a note that said: *We would love to show you a good time.*

As Jane read the note, her body reacted. She loved guys in uniform and was so turned on by the idea of being with the two hot officers. Unfortunately, she had already made plans with the manager who Craig was expecting her to hook up with. *Ugh, what a shame,* she thought.

The manager turned out to be a mediocre lover and the sex was disappointing. She left quite unsatisfied. Walking back to her own room, Jane noticed the piece of paper in her pocket with the salacious note and the officers' room number on it. Feeling like there was nothing to lose, Jane knocked on the soldiers' door and wound up having a fantastic unexpected experience with the two of them. Fucking three guys in one evening blew Craig's mind. From that night on, every time they drove past that hotel together, they exchanged a smirk.

Her Naughty Forties

After leaving the military, Craig married Jane and with the addition of a baby, their crazy sex life was put on hold. The best they could do was to replace the loss of new experiences by the retelling of the old ones for their arousal. It continued like this for several years while they raised their child, and Criag focused on pushing his successful professional career along. His cuckolding fantasies seemed to be in the past . . . until Jane hit forty and met Laura.

Jane quickly developed a close connection to Laura, who was in the process of getting divorced. At first, the hangouts were quite tame, but after three or four times together, the ladies loosened up. Jane would come home and tell Craig how impressed she was watching her brazen friend chat up random guys at the bar. Seeing the potential for fun, Craig pushed Jane to join her friend in the flirting while being the wingwoman.

While he was in London for a work convention, Craig was startled awake when his phone rang at 2 a.m. Upon answering the call from his wife, he realized the line was open and heard Jane talking to Laura in a cab about the two guys they had just been hanging out with.

"Holy shit, they were so fucking hot!"

Laura agreed that their bodies were amazingly fit and admitted she was really turned on by their attention. The ladies were giggling hysterically at the conversation when Laura's tone shifted from playful gossip to genuine curiosity. She worried what Craig was feeling by hearing all this, but Jane assured her that this was something Craig was into. Once Laura knew Jane had free reign to play as much as she wanted, a door was opened, and together the two friends willingly stepped through it.

Each time they went out, Laura promised Craig she would show Jane a good time. She assured him guys would be drooling all over his sexy wife. Soon though, the flirting escalated to more risqué antics. The next time Craig's phone rang in the middle of the night, he assumed they needed a ride home from the nightclub, but instead, he noticed the line was just open. Muffled noises and moans were all he could hear. He quickly realized he was listening to his wife getting fucked. Jane was putting on quite a show for him. Craig's fantasies were finally coming to fruition, and he couldn't have been more elated.

"Yes! Give me that big Black cock baby!"

The sheer ecstasy in her voice made Craig instantly erect. Then to his astonishment, he heard a second male voice in the background, telling her how amazing her ass looked and how tight her pussy felt. Craig closed his eyes and listened carefully as he tried to envision the image of his beautiful wife being taken on both ends by two strong Black men.

When Jane walked through the door a few hours later, she had an epic look of satisfaction. Wanting to be reclaimed, she instructed him to remove her panties and lay down. Her warm thighs felt heavenly wrapped around his cheeks as she straddled his face.

As he feasted on her, she described in detail how she had hooked up with a famous UK athlete and his trainer. How their muscular bodies, impressive stamina, and big cocks—so much bigger than Craig's—had pleasured her. He was in heaven with her sitting on his face and hearing about how many times she orgasmed from the other men. How she couldn't wait to see them again.

The ladies double-dated with them several more times over the next few months, and Craig listened in each time. Sometimes, the eavesdropping sessions were so intense that he couldn't control himself and came all over the place while he listened to the wild sex. It started to become a problem since by the time Jane got back from her frolics with Laura and the men, Craig wasn't able to fulfill his reclaiming duties. Craig realized he needed a chastity device to make sure he would be able to fully please his wife when she got home.

When he shared the idea with Jane, she loved it. As caging became an important part of their kink connection, she told Laura that she was locking him up for the night. The trio developed an erotic routine where Craig dropped them off, opened the doors for them, and kissed Jane goodbye. Laura, who truly enjoyed messing with him, always mockingly tapped his restrained crotch before leaving. She also taunted him throughout the night by sending photos from their escapades. It drove Craig wild with desire. So much so, that they decided to explore humiliation in addition to the teasing and denial. Instead of just knowing his wife had been intimate with another man, he wanted to be involved.

The next time Jane and Laura went out, the plan was for Craig to be present at the start of the evening, so he could meet the girls and their dates and fulfill cuck duties in person. He could only imagine what the men thought as Jane bossed him around like a servant. She tousled his hair and ordered him to be a good hubby. As the four of them sat in the living room, he obediently followed all her instructions to serve them whatever they wanted. If what they wanted wasn't in the house, she sent him to the store to get it for them.

It was hot to see another man with his arms around his wife and he felt like the spare wheel in his relationship. After he drove them to a hotel, she sent him home and the real party started. The two ladies spent all night fucking the two men in all kinds of positions and configurations, while Craig listened to the entire thing on his phone. When Craig dutifully picked them up around 10 a.m. the next morning, both had massive smiles plastered to their faces and told him how well they had been satisfied by the two men.

"I told you I would take care of her," Laura said as she patted him on the head condescendingly.

Craig and Jane were having a blast. Their kinks were so symbiotic. They not only loved each other, but truly appreciated each other. They were always looking for new ways to take it up a notch and decided to create a sex bucket list for Jane. By completing a task, like making out with a stranger, getting fingered in public, giving a blow job in an odd location, or getting fucked in certain ways, she would earn points redeemable for prizes. Gifts ranged from a pair of Louboutins, a trip to New York, and even a BMW convertible.

One night, Jane rang Craig from the club, and amidst the blaring music, he could hear part of her conversation: "Oh god, please finger me right now!"

Craig got as hard as he could in his chastity device as he heard a bucket list item being checked off, when the phone call abruptly disconnected. It was torture as he waited for her to return home and report her activities to him. As usual, Jane strutted through the front door and wasted no time mounting his face. She told him after some playful interaction at the club with the guy and his friend, she and Laura decide to take them out to the alley behind the building. First Jane dropped to her knees, unzipped the first guy's pants, and blew the young stud while his friend filmed. Then his friend passionately pushed Jane up against the wall, lifted her skirt, and fucked her while Laura cheered her on.

Craig was so proud of his hotwife's accomplishment that he took her on a shopping spree the very next day. As he sat on the plush couch in the high-end store, sipping on sparkling water, Craig lovingly watched his wife try on gorgeous dress after gorgeous dress. Seeing her happy and beautiful filled Craig with so much joy. When one of the sales associates commented to him that he had one special woman there, he smiled and thought, *You have no idea.*

All Good Things Come to an End

For a few years Craig lived out his wildest cuckolding fantasies. It was a dream come true. But unfortunately, Jane's bestie eventually settled down into a serious relationship, and their salacious stretch ended. Without her slutty sidekick in tow, Jane no longer wanted to go out at night to bars or indulge in those kinds of adventures. Doing it alone just didn't have the same appeal to her. She knew it was what Craig wanted but she could no longer honestly fulfill the fantasies, and authenticity in their relationship was of paramount importance to both of them. Torn between his desires and his love for his wife to live as she wanted, he did occasionally try to reintroduce the idea but to no avail.

Currently, Craig and Jane still have a great sex life. They frequently hit up hotels to fuck each other while reminiscing about old escapades. Jane lovingly humors his cuck cravings by riding his face as she recounts more untold filthy stories from her "naughty forties" past. Craig also replays any one of the collection of memories he has burned into his brain when he needs a thrill. Although the element of hotwifing is no longer a part of their marriage, to this day, Jane still remains the love of his life.

Based on episode

382 - Craig Is a True Cuckold, and He Married the Ultimate Hotwife

CONFESSION XVII: ABBY

Abby was twenty-two years old and still dating the first guy she ever had sex with. Little did they know when they first hooked up that eventually they would also both be hooking up with her best friend who happened to be a trans man. So how did they all wind up in a steamy hot throuple?

From a very early age, Abby always knew she was highly sexual, often describing her young self as a "horny little beast." Her family was pretty relaxed about sex too. Growing up, word around town was that her dad was a "manwhore." She realized this first-hand when at thirteen, she walked in on him having sex with one of her schoolteachers. Apparently, he was having sex with lots of different women, and it wasn't something he hid or was ashamed of.

Becoming Kinky

A couple of years later Abby met her boyfriend. They were both virgins and after losing their virginity to each other, Abby, "the horny little beast," rolled over and immediately declared: "I want to have sex every single day."

Her boyfriend, who was a lot less horny than she was, wasn't sure he was up to the task, but promised to try. Eager to have more than just basic, vanilla sex, Abby started opening up to her boyfriend about all the kinky things she was interested in trying. She admitted she was curious about cuffs and being restrained, and that she frequently watched bondage videos. When she asked him what kind of videos he liked to watch, his response surprised her.

"I just go to Pornhub and watch whatever comes up."

Abby couldn't believe it and pushed him harder. She knew there had to be something out of the ordinary that he was secretly into. With further prodding he confessed that he got turned on watching anime if the women were drawn with big thighs. He loved to see them dressed up in costumes, specifically when they wore tights and pantyhose. He fantasized about what it would feel like to touch their big thighs in pantyhose and to feel the restriction of their skin in the fabric. His fantasy was to have his face between Abby's thighs while she wore a pair. As it turned out, Abby's prodding had helped her boyfriend realize he had a full-fledged pantyhose fetish.

Abby was super excited to have found something nonvanilla in her otherwise vanilla boyfriend and thought to herself *I can work with this*. With her newfound knowledge of her boyfriend's fetish, she started incorporating pantyhose and costumes into their everyday life and took on the role of his submissive. They set up a routine: she would come home from work, throw on a maid's outfit with a pair of tights, and start cleaning up around the house. Then it was game on. He was allowed to bend her over, rip off her tights, and fuck her anytime he wanted until it was time for bed.

Although Abby enjoyed being a sub, she also found herself extremely turned on by femdom porn. Soon she decided to switch things up and started wearing thigh-highs and leather to mimic the outfits she saw the women in the videos wearing. When she switched to being the Domme, her boyfriend quickly took to being the sub and he even started cleaning the house himself to please her. As masculine as her boyfriend was, his submissive side turned her on too. Abby and her boyfriend found they were both equally into being the Dom/Domme, and the sub, and they switched roles often.

At times, he would be the dominant one. There were days he would tie her up, and then insert a vibrator inside her and leave her there for hours at a time. Other times she would return the favor by tying him up, placing a vibrator right on his dick, and leaving him there for hours.

One time, Abby tied him up in his room for an entire day. She spent that whole day teasing and denying him. She would randomly walk in, spank him, and then she'd walk out, leaving him wanting more. She did it over and over again until he couldn't take it anymore. She then started playing with his cock, touching it until he came, and then left him there unable to clean up. She repeated the entire process over and over and wound up giving him five massive orgasms that day.

When she told her boyfriend that she had a pegging fantasy, she got her first pushback. He wasn't even comfortable having a finger anywhere near his asshole, and so he definitely wasn't into having her shove a dildo up his ass. But knowing he was open-minded at his core, she continued to gently push the topic. Eventually he agreed to let her use a butt plug on him, and to both of their surprise, he wound up having his very first prostate orgasm. He could barely walk afterward and described it as the most mind-shattering orgasm he had ever had.

After about a year of using the butt plug, he finally agreed to let her peg him. They started the night off with butt plug play to slowly stretch him out. After some time, Abby added her finger, and then a bigger butt plug. Slowly she worked the bigger plug in and out of him until she could tell he was turned on and super relaxed. Abby then forced him to his knees, tied his hands behind his back, and bent him over. She was super turned on as she got behind him and strapped on her dildo.

She positioned the strap-on against him and gently pushed the head in first. As he relaxed into it, she put both hands on his hips and slowly pulled him in until the dildo was all the way in. At first, she moved in and out slowly until she could tell he wanted it faster.

As she continued to peg him, she reached around and started to jerk him off at the same time. She continued for a while and though he never finished while she was pegging him, he really enjoyed the experience. Abby fucking loved it.

From Couple to Throuple

About eight years earlier, Abby had met a guy who would become her best friend. He was just starting his transition from female to male and they immediately clicked. Over the years, even though Abby always thought he was superhot, they had never hooked up. It was only when Abby and her boyfriend started experimenting that Abby started fantasizing about her best friend in a sexual way.

Eventually she decided to admit that she was into him and to her surprise he was too. Unfortunately, when she told her boyfriend about their attraction and asked if it was okay for them to hook up, he wasn't into it. He didn't want her hooking up with other guys. Not to be deterred, Abby started bringing her best friend around her boyfriend all the time. She was hoping that if they grew to be friends, her boyfriend would grow more comfortable with the idea and change his mind.

And that's exactly what happened. Her boyfriend and best friend became closer, and he eventually gave them a free pass to hook up without him. But he had a few rules he wanted Abby to follow: he was okay with them fingering each other and using a strap-on, but he wasn't okay with kissing and oral sex. Abby agreed and quickly told her friend the good news.

The following week she showed up at her friend's house excited to hook up. The plan was to take some naughty photos of Abby by the creek near his house. It was the first time her friend was seeing her naked and as Abby stripped down, she could tell her friend was aroused, as was Abby. Being outside, naked, in front of someone so close to her was a total turn-on. The minute they were finished and back in his house, her friend blurted out: "I'm really horny."

Abby was really horny too, and they both began taking their clothes off. Her best friend laid down on the bed, secured his strap-on, and instructed Abby to get on top of him and ride it. As Abby rode his strap-on she pressed a vibrator on her clit until she had the best orgasm she'd ever had. The whole thing was superhot and they captured it all on video. Abby still watches that video to this day.

When Abby got home, she was dying to tell her boyfriend all about it and show him the video, but he didn't want to see or hear the details. He was just happy that she had a good time and told her that if she wanted to do it again, he'd totally be okay with it.

The very next weekend the best friend came over to their house, and they all decided to do shrooms together. It ended up being a powerful bonding experience between the three of them. Abby was happy because it brought her best friend and her boyfriend closer in a way they hadn't been before, and they even started talking about what it would be like if the two of them were to have sex together. Abby couldn't believe that her boyfriend was open to it and was turned on by all the thought of the three of them possibly hooking up.

Abby's birthday was the following week, and they invited the best friend over to celebrate with them. While the three of them were hanging out, Abby's boyfriend let the words slip out: "I want to see you guys kiss."

They all went into the bedroom together and with the kissing rule apparently off the table, Abby and her best friend started making out right in front of him. Abby could tell her boyfriend was super turned on just watching them, but she wanted him to join in. Abby's best friend had always had a fantasy of a man finishing inside his pussy and so they asked Abby's boyfriend if he was down to fuck him. Her boyfriend was okay with it but didn't think he would be able to finish inside of him while looking at his facial hair.

Determined to make her best friend's fantasy come true, Abby sat on her boyfriend's face so he couldn't see anything. And that totally worked for him. As the best friend started riding her boyfriend's cock, Abby started grinding her hips onto her boyfriend's face. As the best friend rode her boyfriend, Abby leaned in and started making out with him at the same time. It was so hot Abby couldn't control herself and quickly came all over her boyfriend's face. The minute she was done coming, her boyfriend came inside her best friend's pussy and then her best friend's climax followed. It was an amazing experience for all three of them.

After that night, all the rules were taken off the table and Abby could do whatever she wanted with her best friend, whenever she wanted to. Sometimes she played alone with him and sometimes the three of them would hook up. Eventually, over time, her boyfriend and best friend decided they wanted to hook up with each other too. The three of them had been joking about her cucking the two of them and so they decided to hook up with each other while Abby watched. Abby set up a lawn chair in the bedroom, grabbed a bag of chips, and watched them fuck. She took pictures and recorded the whole experience. Although being the cuck wasn't a big turn-on for her, she still enjoyed herself. It was highly entertaining watching two people fuck in front of her, something she had never seen live before.

Although Abby loves the throuple she has going on with her boyfriend and her best friend, it really only works because her best friend hasn't had his bottom surgery yet. He still has a biologically female lower half, and that is what Abby's most into. Abby recently realized she's way more into girls than guys and told her boyfriend that if they ever broke up, she'd only date women. With her best friend's bottom surgery looming in the future, they're currently on the hunt for a cisgender female to join them in the bedroom.

Even More Exploration

Abby's boyfriend one day admitted to her that he was interested in the idea of public sex. Something about them being seen and/or caught really turned him on and the thought of it kind of turned Abby on too. They started out having sex in his truck by the side of the road while other cars went by, and it drove him wild. So much so that every time they did it, he would be horned up and all over her for weeks afterward. As they got braver, they started pushing the boundaries even further. One time, in the middle of the afternoon while alone at a public picnic spot in their hometown, they decided to get it on.

Abby's boyfriend instructed her to strip down out of her clothes, and soon she was standing there, totally naked in the middle of the picnic area in broad daylight. Completely aroused, her boyfriend turned her around, bent her over a picnic table, and started fucking her. Eventually he pulled out of her pussy and then slowly began fucking her in the ass right there in the park. She immediately took one of her hands and started rubbing her clit until they both came.

That was hot as fuck, she thought as she started to put herself back together.

Just as they were finished putting their clothes on, a family walked into the picnic area to have their lunch. As they sat down on the very table they had just been fucking on, Abby couldn't help but laugh.

Having experienced being an exhibitionist Abby has recently found that she really enjoys being watched online and has started posting her sexcapades on OnlyFans. She's still very into dressing up for her boyfriend and will frequently post videos of her in costumes, as well as pics of her in lingerie and bondage photos. She also posts videos of her and her best friend hooking up, her and her boyfriend hooking up, as well as the three of them hooking up. Both her boyfriend and her best friend are totally cool with being featured in her videos, and she loves taping and sharing their content with others.

Currently Abby is still on the hunt for a unicorn. She really wants her boyfriend to hook up with other women outside of their relationship and tell her about it, but as of now it hasn't happened yet. Abby and her boyfriend love exploring and being in an open relationship. And over communicating about their wants, needs, and desires is what makes it all work for them. The icing on the cake is that they still have her best friend exploring with them too.

Based on episode

993 - Abby and Her BF are In a Poly Throuple with a Trans Man

ACKNOWLEDGMENTS

A special thanks first and foremost to my callers and my listeners. Without them there would be no show, no killer stories, and therefore, no book. I would like to thank, in no particular order, Adam Darrow, Casey Donatello, Mike Lewis, and Lexi Silver for helping me write this book as well as SDC.com for providing the Sexxxy Terms You Need to Know. I also want to thank Scott Kaufman and Conan Smith at Don Buchwald Agency as well as Jarred Wesifeld, Ashley Calvano, and Start Romance for being so open-minded and cool enough to put these true stories out there. Lastly, thanks to my son for just existing.

ABOUT THE AUTHOR

Kathy Kay is a content creator and host who started the highly acclaimed *Strictly Anonymous Confessions* podcast over a decade ago, amassing over one thousand episodes. Driven by an innate sense of curiosity, a genuine desire to help people with their problems, and an unwavering commitment to nonjudgmental support, Kay embarked on this remarkable podcasting journey. One interesting aspect of Kathy's bio lies in her own secret life—her podcast. With an air of intrigue, she has successfully maintained anonymity, concealing her identity from not only her listeners but also her own family and closest friends. This carefully crafted mystique adds a unique allure to the Strictly Anonymous Confessions brand that she has built over the years. Drawing from her background in entertainment as a talent booker, Kay possesses a tenacious work ethic and an uncanny ability to accomplish goals with unwavering determination. These qualities have been instrumental in consistently building her podcast to secure a top position on the iTunes and Spotify charts, all while remaining anonymous.